Contraceptive Research, Introduction, and Use

Lessons from Norplant

Polly F. Harrison and Allan Rosenfield, *Editors*

Subcommittee for Workshop on Implant Contraceptives:
An Illuminating Case Study in Current
Dilemmas and Possibilities

Committee on Contraceptive Research and Development

Division of Health Sciences Policy

INSTITUTE OF MEDICINE

NATIONAL ACADEMY PRESS
Washington, D.C. 1998

NATIONAL ACADEMY PRESS • 2101 Constitution Avenue, N.W. • Washington, D.C. 20418

NOTICE: The project that is the subject of this report was approved by the Governing Board of the National Research Council, whose members are drawn from the councils of the National Academy of Sciences, the National Academy of Engineering, and the Institute of Medicine. The members of the committee responsible for the report were chosen for their special competences and with regard for appropriate balance. This report has been reviewed by a group other than the authors according to procedures approved by a Report Review Committee consisting of members of the National Academy of Sciences, the National Academy of Engineering, and the Institute of Medicine.

The Institute of Medicine was chartered in 1970 by the National Academy of Sciences to enlist distinguished members of the appropriate professions in the examination of policy matters pertaining to the health of the public. In this, the Institute acts under both the Academy's 1863 congressional charter responsibility to be an adviser to the federal government and its own initiative in identifying issues of medical care, research, and education. Dr. Kenneth I. Shine is president of the Institute of Medicine.

This study was supported by a grant from the Henry J. Kaiser Family Foundation, Menlo Park, California. The views presented in this report are those of the Committee on Contraceptive Research and Development and are not necessarily those of the funding organization.

International Standard Book No. 0-309-05985-2

Additional copies of *Contraceptive Research, Introduction, and Use: Lessons from Norplant*, are available for sale from the National Academy Press, Box 285, 2101 Constitution Avenue, N.W., Washington, DC 20055; Call (800) 624-6242 or (202) 334-3313 (in the Washington metropolitan area), or visit the NAP's on-line bookstore at **http://www.nap.edu**.

For more information about the Institute of Medicine, visit the IOM home page at **http://www2.nas.edu/iom**.

Copyright 1998 by the National Academy of Sciences. All rights reserved.

Printed in the United States of America

SUBCOMMITTEE FOR WORKSHOP ON IMPLANT CONTRACEPTIVES

Allan Rosenfield[*] (*Chair*), Dean, School of Public Health, Columbia University
Hedia Belhadj-El Ghouayel, Deputy to the Director, Division for Arab States and Europe, United Nations Population Fund, New York
Nancy L. Buc, Partner, Buc & Beardsley, Washington, D.C.
Rebecca J. Cook, Professor, Faculty of Law, University of Toronto
Richard H. Douglas, Vice President, Corporate Development, Genzyme Corporation, Boston
Donald Patrick McDonnell, Associate Professor of Pharmacology, Duke University Medical Center
David C. Mowery, Professor of Business and Public Policy, Walter A. Haas School of Business, University of California at Berkeley
Judy Norsigian, Co-director, Boston Women's Health Book Collective

Study Staff

Polly F. Harrison, Senior Study Director
Gretchen Ganzle Kidder, Research Assistant
Christina Thacker, Project Assistant

Division Staff

Valerie P. Setlow, Director
Linda DePugh, Administrative Assistant
Jamaine Tinker, Financial Associate

---

[*]Institute of Medicine member.

COMMITTEE ON CONTRACEPTIVE RESEARCH AND DEVELOPMENT

Allan Rosenfield[*] (*Chair*), Dean, School of Public Health, Columbia University
Hedia Belhadj El Ghouayel, Deputy to the Director, Division for Arab States and Europe, United Nations Population Fund, New York
Donald D. Brown,[†] Director, Department of Embryology, Carnegie Institute of Washington, Baltimore, Maryland
Nancy L. Buc, Partner, Buc & Beardsley, Washington, D.C.
Peter F. Carpenter, Founder/Director, Mission and Values Institute, Visiting Scholar, Center for Biomedical Ethics, Stanford University
Willard Cates, Jr., Corporate Director of Medical Affairs, Family Health International, Research Triangle Park, North Carolina
Rebecca J. Cook, Professor, Faculty of Law, University of Toronto
Horacio B. Croxatto, Professor, Instituto Chilena de Medicina Reproductiva, Santiago, Chile
Richard H. Douglas, Vice President, Corporate Development, Genzyme Corporation, Boston
Michael J. K. Harper, Professor, Department of Obstetrics and Gynecology, Eastern Virginia Medical School
Donald Patrick McDonnell, Associate Professor of Pharmacology, Duke University Medical Center
David C. Mowery, Professor of Business and Public Policy, Walter A. Haas School of Business, University of California at Berkeley
Judy Norsigian, Co-director, Boston Women's Health Book Collective
Sandra Panem, Managing Partner, Vector Fund Management, Vector Securities International, Deerfield, Illinois
Bennett M. Shapiro, Executive Vice President, Worldwide Basic Research, Merck Research Laboratories, Rahway, New Jersey
Wylie Vale,[†] Professor, The Clayton Foundation Laboratories for Peptide Biology, The Salk Institute, La Jolla, California
Bai-ge Zhao, Director, Shanghai Institute of Planned Parenthood Research

---

[*]Institute of Medicine member.
[†]National Academy of Sciences member.

Acknowledgments

This document reports the proceedings of a workshop that depended for any useful outcome not just on the knowledge and experience of its participants but on their willingness to engage in flexible and open dialogue. Much appreciation is owed to:

- presenters James Anderson, David Archer, Marie Bass, Paul Blumenthal, Ward Cates, Jacqueline Darroch, Angela Davey, Andrew Davidson, Lynne Gaffikin, Michael Green, Debra Kalmuss, Helen Koo, Preston Marx, Olav Meirik, Noel Rose, Ruth Simmons, Irving Sivin, Felicia Stewart, and Paul Van Look;
- panelists Martha Katz, Ruth Macklin, Ellen Moskowitz, Cynthia Pearson, Julia Scott, and Marian Secundy, and
- all participants, whose expertise and commitment contributed so constructively to advancing understanding of a persistently difficult subject.

As small as this document is, much work went into its preparation. For that we thank our project staff Christina Thacker and Gretchen Kidder, who handled the workshop logistics, drafted the presentation summaries, and prepared this document for the press; Claudia Carl, who shepherded the report through review; Michael Edington, who helped with its editing and publication; and Valerie Setlow, who was unfailingly helpful in many ways.

We also offer our thanks to the subcommittee for its willingness to continue membership on the Committee on Contraceptive Research and Development in order to encompass this activity.

Finally, we thank the Henry J. Kaiser Family Foundation for its support, patience, and unflagging conviction that this is a very important topic.

To all, our gratitude is very great and most sincere.

Allan Rosenfield, *Chair*
Polly F. Harrison, *Senior Study Director*

Contents

1 INTRODUCTION 1

2 WORKSHOP REPORT 3
   Efficacy and Safety, 3
      Efficacy, 3
      Safety, 4
   Who Uses Norplant and How, 9
      User Populations, 9
      Method Continuation and Discontinuation, 11
      Side Effects as Factors, 12
      User Satisfaction, 13
      Barriers to Discontinuation, 18
   Insertion and Removal: Experience and Implications, 23
      Technical Aspects, 23
      Case Experiences, 23
      Rates of Complicated Removals, 25
      Implications, 25
   Consumer Perspectives, 27
      Communication and Quality of Care, 27
      Informed Decision-Making, 28
      Consumer Involvement, 31
   New Approaches, 31
      Reproductive Health Technologies Project's "Boom and Bust Initiative," 32
      The WHO Strategic Approach to Contraceptive Introduction, 32
      A "Government Standards Defense," 34

3 WORKSHOP SUMMARY AND ANALYSIS 37

Data Review, 38
    Efficacy, 38
    Safety, 38
    User Profiles, 39
    Side Effects, 39
    Continuation and Discontinuation, 39
    User Satisfaction, 40
    Postmarketing Surveillance, 40
    Cost-Effectiveness, 41

Lessons Learned, 41

Next Steps: Areas for Consideration and Action, 44
    Areas for Strengthening or Expansion, 44
    Areas for New Initiative, 47

Final Comment, 49

APPENDIXES

A   Presentation Summaries, 59
B   Norplant: Historical Background, 107
C   Workshop Agenda, 115

1

Introduction

In late 1996, the Institute of Medicine's (IOM) Committee on Contraceptive Research and Development completed a major study of the state of contraceptive science, the need for new contraceptives, and factors helping or hindering response to that need.[1] As part of its work, the committee reviewed case histories of experience with the development and introduction of new contraceptives, including a brief review of the contraceptive implant, Norplant®. The committee believed that the Norplant experience echoed critical elements in the history of several other contraceptives and that a detailed analysis of that experience would be particularly instructive. As the first real contraceptive innovation in over two decades and as a long-acting method requiring clinical intervention for application and removal, the method raised an especially wide range of issues that could offer valuable lessons about the barriers and problems to be addressed if other new technologies are to enter the contraceptive marketplace.

Thus, in April 1997, a subcommittee of that original study committee convened a workshop, *Implant Contraceptives: An Illuminating Case Study in Current Dilemmas and Possibilities*.[2] Its objectives were to: (1) review newly available data on Norplant's efficacy, safety, and use; (2) extract lessons from presentations on diverse aspects of the method's development, introduction, use, and market experience; and, (3) explore approaches to developing and introducing new contraceptives based on learning from that experience.

The workshop consisted of 17 formal presentations; two organized dialogues, one on consumer perspectives, the other on new strategies for developing and introducing new contraceptive technologies; and extensive discussion among subcommittee members, presenters, and invited participants on the information presented and its implications. The subcommittee met in executive session after adjournment to analyze the workshop proceedings and develop a list of lessons and points for further consideration or action.

The report is organized in the following manner: The first section reviews the major points in the workshop presentations and dialogues, concluding with a summation of the principal lessons they provided and the areas of action most urgently suggested for the future. It is followed by three appendixes and detailed endnotes. Appendix A contains abstracts of the 15 formal presentations in a common format. Appendix B presents background material on the technology and a chronology of its development and market experience. Appendix C provides the workshop agenda and list of participants. The endnotes consist of references made by presenters and other information deemed necessary to support and clarify the text.

2

Workshop Report

EFFICACY AND SAFETY

The first workshop task was to review two fundamental matters: Norplant's efficacy and its safety. These issues were addressed in a series of six presentations,[*] each based on accumulated experience and on fresh analysis of new data:

- the 5-year Postmarketing Surveillance of Norplant conducted by the World Health Organization's (WHO) Special Program for Research, Development, and Research Training in Human Reproduction (WHO/HRP), with the Population Council and Family Health International (FHI) (*Presentation 1*)
- 5-year Population Council studies of women using Norplant and women using the two-rod levonorgestrel implant system (LNG ROD) (*Presentation 2*)
- analyses of putative association between silicone and systemic disease (*Presentations 3, 4*)
- analyses of relevance of reports on the effect of progesterone-induced changes on viral infectivity in a monkey model (*Presentations 5, 6*).

Efficacy

The workshop presentations on the Postmarketing Surveillance led by WHO/HRP and on the Population Council studies confirmed what has been found in all long-term studies of Norplant since 1980[3]—that is, that its contraceptive efficacy is very high and that return of fertility after removal of the implant is rapid.

---

[*]See Appendix A, *Presentations 1* (Meirik), *2* (Sivin), *3* (Rose), *4* (Anderson), *5* (Marx), and *6* (Cates).

The purpose of the Postmarketing Surveillance was to study, over a 5-year period, major short- to medium-term side effects of Norplant not identified in clinical trials. The Surveillance followed a sample of 7,977 women for 5 years (a total of 33,627 woman-years) and found a pregnancy rate of 0.23 per 100 woman-years. For purposes of comparison, the Surveillance also followed two control groups: women who had chosen the copper-bearing intrauterine device (IUD) and women who had chosen tubal ligation. The pregnancy rates for these two groups were 0.80 and 0.15 per 100 woman-years, respectively.

The Population Council studies, undertaken to gather data for Food and Drug Administration (FDA) approval of the two-rod implant and to obtain additional information for revision of Norplant's labeling, found similarly high efficacy. In studies between 1990 and 1996 of 2,798 women in seven countries, the Council found that Norplant and the LNG ROD had similar hormonal release rates and virtually indistinguishable pregnancy rates. The cumulative 5-year pregnancy rate for the samples analyzed collectively was 1.1 per 100 woman-years.

Table 2-1, provided to the subcommittee after the workshop as additional detail for purposes of comparison, presents data on first-year and 5-year pregnancy rates for Norplant and the LNG ROD from studies in 14 countries. The evidence from those studies and from the new data presented at the workshop was that both Norplant and two-rod levonorgestrel implant system are highly efficacious, with failure rates under 1 percent per year, thus providing reversible contraceptive protection essentially equal to that of permanent methods—tubal ligation and vasectomy.

Safety

Like all hormonal contraceptives, Norplant, even though it is well tolerated by many women, is associated with adverse reactions or events.[4] These are described in the prescribing information for providers and in patient labeling, both of which continue to be updated as new data become available. Of greatest concern are potential medical complications that pose serious risks to the health of the user. The Postmarketing Surveillance analysis refers to these as "major health-related events," defined as including the following: all pregnancies, all deaths, and all complications that are potentially life-threatening, require hospitalization or at least 1 month of convalescence, leave long-term sequelae, and/or require long-term medication. A second category comprises "significant health-related problems" that may affect quality of life; these were defined as virtually anything except common colds and minor injuries. Although not life-threatening, the problems in this category may range from tolerable to annoying for some women, from distressing to intolerable for others.

TABLE 2-1 First-Year and Five-Year Pregnancy Rates and Continuation Rates for Contraceptive Implants[5]

Method, Country	Reference	N	First-Year Rates		Five-Year Rates	
			Pregnancy	Continuation	Pregnancy	Continuation
Norplant[g]						
Bangladesh	Akhter, 1993	600	0.0	93.9	0.0	41.2
Chile	Diaz, 1982	101	0.0	88.0	0.0	54.0
China	Gu, 1994	10,718	0.1	94.1	1.5	72.1
Dominican Republic	Sivin, 1988	1,009	0.2	79.0	3.5	25.0
Egypt	Salah, 1987	250	1.3	90.0	1.6*	58.0
Indonesia	Affandi, 1987	437	0.0	96.5	1.8	78.2
Indonesia	Noerpramana, 1995	170	0.0	97.6	0.0	90.0
Nepal	Grubb, 1995	1,203	0.5	89.0	0.8	56.4
Philippines	Grubb, 1995	300	0.0	95.3	1.7	64.2
Scandinavia	Sivin, 1988	377	0.0	76.0	2.7	33.0
Singapore	Singh, 1992	100	0.0	97.0	0.0	59.7
Sri Lanka	Grubb, 1995	755	0.4	95.6	0.6	45.5
Thailand	Chompootaweep, 1996	308	0.0	97.6	4.2	71.0
United States	Sivin, 1988	355	0.0	82.0	≥ 5.2	≤ 44.0
United States	Frank, 1993	1,253	0.2	87.1	NA	NA
United States	Crosby, 1993	2,358	0.0	92.6	NA	NA
U.S. teenagers	Cullins, 1994	136	0.0	92.0	NA	NA
U.S. adults	Cullins, 1994	542	0.0	90.0	NA	NA
United Kingdom	Peers, 1996	2,126	0.0	85.2	NA	NA
LNG ROD						
China	Gu, 1994	1,208	0.1	94.3	0.6	65.3
India	ICMR, 1993	1,466	0.0	88.0	0.8	57.9
Singapore	Singh, 1992	100	0.0	95.0	0.0	62.0

*Multiple decrement rate.

Major Health-Related Events

Both the Postmarketing Surveillance of Norplant and the 1990–1996 Population Council studies of Norplant and the LNG ROD found serious adverse events to be rare among implant users over 5 years of study. The overall mortality rate for the Population Council samples at 5 years after initiating levonorgestrel implant use was 1.1 per 10,000 woman-years of observation, well below the expected rate. Hospitalization rates for these study samples were compared with two sets of control data (a 1995 U.S. hospital discharge survey and a study in the United Kingdom by Martin Vessey in 1976), and proved to be substantially below the hospitalization rates for both those data sets. The Postmarketing Surveillance found 9 deaths in 33,627 woman-years of Norplant use; there were no differences in the overall mortality rates among women using Norplant, women using the IUD, and women who had opted for sterilization.

Nor did the Surveillance identify significant long-term morbidity. Norplant users were found to be at very low risk of ectopic pregnancy, 0.03 per 100 woman-years on average, compared to a rate of 0.19 per 100 woman-years for non-contracepting women.[6] The Surveillance data were also described as reassuring with respect to cardiovascular disease, stroke, gallbladder disease, neoplastic disease, and anemias. Frequencies of systemic lupus erythematosus and collagen diseases, about which questions had been raised in connection with Norplant, were far too low to permit any conclusions. Diagnosis of hypertension was somewhat higher in Norplant users compared to IUD users and sterilized women.

Significant Health-Related Problems

The Surveillance analysis included in this category mood disturbances, anxiety, and depression; migraine or other headaches; and visual disturbances. While there initially seemed to be higher incidence of visual disturbances in Norplant users, closer scrutiny revealed no causal relationships. Mood disturbances were recorded more frequently among Norplant users than among IUD users, but their incidence was similar to that generally found with other hormonal methods of contraception. In fact, the presenter commented, noting that the observation was likely to be controversial, that Norplant appears to produce patterns of adverse effects very similar to those of combined oral contraceptives (COCs).

The noteworthy exception is changes in menstrual patterns, of which the most important are prolonged or irregular menstrual flow or increased bleeding. These changes do seem to be more commonly associated with Norplant than with COCs, although firm conclusions in that regard are constrained by lack of explicitly comparative data. The Emory/Columbia/CMC study that is discussed in greater detail below reported that, in its sample of U.S. women, fewer of the women using oral contraceptives experienced menstrual side effects, although a substantial majority of those women had at least one such experience. Women using Norplant were considerably more likely to experience longer periods, irregular cycles, and heavier bleeding than those using either the pill or Depo-Provera.

As with all hormonal methods, Norplant is unsuitable for some women and the contraindications involved are detailed in its labeling. The workshop presentations concurred that, in the settings where these studies were carried out, the evidence from five years of follow-up was that the method had proved to be not only highly effective but safe and well-tolerated. There was also agreement that the Postmarketing Surveillance of Norplant was valuable not only as a source of knowledge on side effects not identified in clinical trials, but as evidence that large-scale, longer-term studies using cohort methodology can now be considered feasible in developing countries.

*Silicone Biocompatibility**

The possibility of association between silicone-/gel-filled breast implants and connective tissue or autoimmune disease has stimulated questions about other implants, including contraceptive implants, that employ other silicone materials.[7] Two workshop presentations (*3* and *4*) addressed this topic from different perspectives. The first reported on studies of the biocompatibility (biological response testing) and inherent characteristics of the filled silicone elastomer or polymer known as "silicone rubber" that is a component of the Norplant implant system. The second reevaluated an earlier study (Rochester [New York] General Hospital)[8] which had raised concerns about the possibility that silicone gel might act as an adjuvant that could potentiate autoimmune disease, concerns subsequently extended to a wider range of silicone implants. The reevaluation first set out to confirm, or not, that silicone gel might act as an adjuvant and, second, to determine whether silicone elastomer of the type used in Norplant might have adjuvant properties.

These analyses made the following points. First, the filler material used in the Norplant tubing is an amorphous silica, not a crystalline silica of the sort that has been associated with pathological problems, and is treated in a way that allows each silica particle to react directly with the polymer chain that holds it within the network structure. Furthermore, it is the silicone polymer, not amorphous silica, that is present at the surface of the tubing, and the surface properties of filled silicone elastomers do not include potential for abrasion.

Second, the biocompatibility studies, which looked at blood protein absorption, inflammatory response, and fibrous capsule formation, suggest that silicone rubber may actually be more biocompatible than several other major biomaterials (dacron, polyethylene, and expanded polytetrafluoroethylene) used in

---

*See Appendix A, *Presentations 3* (Rose) and *4* (Anderson).

other implants. Any material that is implanted, in effect, creates an injury which then produces an inflammatory response; this local foreign-body reaction is typically present at all biomaterial or medical device prosthetic interfaces with tissue; Norplant is not distinctive in this regard.

Third, the silicone gel in breast implants is not the same, chemically or biologically, as the silicone rubber used in Norplant, and there is no indication that that elastomer is implicated in immunological response. Experiments in rat and mouse models used a standard adjuvant (Freund's) as the control, and a silicone oil/gel combination combined with a foreign substance (bovine serum albumen [BSA]) that contained large and small particles of silicone elastomer of the type used in Norplant. While a marked local inflammatory response resulted, neither the large nor small particles potentiated antibody response, indicating that the presence of an inflammatory response did not entail any adjuvant activity. Therefore, were any silicone elastomer particulates to become detached from the Norplant implant, they would produce no adjuvant effect and, consequently, no risk of developing autoimmune disease associated with that biomaterial.

In sum, the Norplant implant system uses amorphous silica rather than the crystalline silica alleged to have been associated with problems, and there is no evidence that this silicone rubber is implicated in any immunologic response, even though there will be an inflammatory reaction, as to any foreign body. The presenters agreed that a matter of great concern, one that could conceivably affect the supply of biomaterial for implant contraceptives, is the current controversy and litigation over silicone products. They noted, furthermore, the much wider and negative effects of that controversy on the supply of polymers and biomaterials needed for medical devices in general, some of which—for example, cerebrospinal fluid shunt systems and pacemaker leads—are essential to life. They referred to those concerns as having precipitated the Biomaterials Access Assurance Act, which became part of the defeated Common Sense Products Liability and Legal Reform Act of 1995, which proposed to protect suppliers from lawsuits in which a company's only role is to provide the raw material.[9]

Progestin Effects on Vaginal HIV Transmission*

Presentation 5 reported on research at the Aaron Diamond AIDS Research Center in a rhesus macaque monkey model developed to investigate the effect of progesterone on vaginal transmission of simian immunodeficiency virus (SIV).[10] Monthly subcutaneous progesterone implants had been found to facilitate the infectivity of cell-free SIV, owing to progesterone-induced changes (basically, thinning of the mucosa) in the monkey's vaginal and cervical epithelium that appeared to reduce anatomic barriers to SIV infection. Future research is planned that will look at differences in susceptibility to infection and the implications of

---

*See Appendix A, *Presentations 5* (Marx) and *6* (Cates).

natural changes in estrogen and progesterone in different phases of the menstrual cycle, as well as the degree of protection afforded by estrogen. More research is also needed on vaginal response to hormones, as well as other monkey studies that would include exploration into cyclic hormonal effects and the effects of progestin use in contraceptives on incidence of SIV infection.

Presentation 6 examined the extent to which these results can be extrapolated to use of Norplant or Depo-Provera in human beings, since SIV is not HIV and since the monkey vagina apparently responds differently to hormones than does the human vagina. Extension of these findings to humans has been limited so far by the fact that epidemiological data and analysis that might cast some light on the subject do not exist at an adequate level of quality or power. Lack of randomized controlled trials, design limitations in most controlled cohort studies, confounding, and small sample sizes were all said to be at issue. A recent effort to draw systematic conclusions from a group of observational studies foundered on these same difficulties and on lack of consistency in critical respects.

Given these basic and clinical research needs, a June 1996 consensus panel at the National Institute of Child Health and Human Development was reported to have concluded that until better human studies become available, the most prudent path will be to reorder clinical management priorities for counseling high-risk clients. The first priority for these clients is to ensure protection from sexually transmitted infections (i.e., through regular condom use and other risk-reduction strategies); optimal protection against conception (i.e., through implant use) becomes second priority. Workshop participants noted that human studies including vaginal biopsies are also being developed and commented that the potential for doing randomized studies in human populations will be both ethically and practically challenging.

WHO USES NORPLANT AND HOW[*]

User Populations

The characteristics of the women in the Postmarketing Surveillance sample differed substantially from country to country (*Presentation 1*). While the majority of Norplant users in that sample were aged 24–35 at time of method adoption, women in the samples in China and Egypt tended to be older at time of adoption than Norplant users in South America and "other Asia" (i.e., Bangladesh, Indonesia, Sri Lanka, and Thailand). In all countries included in the Surveillance, women opting for sterilization had less education than those opting for either an IUD or Norplant, and women opting for Norplant had less education than IUD users; the exception to the latter was South America, where IUD and Norplant users had similar educational levels.

---

[*]See Appendix A, *Presentations 1* (Meirik), *7* (Darroch), *8* (Kalmuss, Davidson), and *9* (Koo).

The most representative picture of who uses Norplant in the United States comes from data, presented at the workshop* and gathered in the 1995 National Survey of Family Growth (NSFG) in a national probability sample of 10,847 women aged 15–44.[11] Of that sample, just 104 women, 1 percent of the total, were current Norplant users; women who had ever used the implant totaled 2 percent.[12] These same overall percentages appeared in the 1996 Ortho Birth Control Studies, also reported in this same presentation.[13] These utilization figures are lower than those found either in developing countries or in Scandinavia where, according to one participant, Norplant's market share was said to run around 3 percent.

Despite limits imposed on analysis by the small number of Norplant users, the NSFG data permit insights into who, as of 1995, was using the method and where it was being obtained. Norplant use was importantly affected by age, Medicaid coverage, parity, and geography, with age the most strongly associated factor. Most women in the NSFG sample who were currently using Norplant were under age 30. Women aged 20–24 were the largest group of users, representing 4 percent of all women using reversible contraceptive methods and a little under 4 percent of all women contracepting. Women aged 15–19 were proportionally the next largest group, followed by women aged 25–29. Women over age 30 accounted for progressively smaller proportions of Norplant users, as increasing numbers appear to opt for sterilization.

Only a very small proportion of women using Norplant had had no children and most had had more than one child. Women on Medicaid were also considerably more likely to use Norplant and younger women, especially those in their early 20s, were more likely to adopt Norplant than women of the same age band who were not on Medicaid. One-third of women using Norplant in 1995 obtained it from a clinic and better than half of those women obtained it from a publicly funded clinic, much smaller proportions than was the case for women using Depo-Provera. Overall, the picture of Norplant users that emerges from the NSFG is of predominantly young, single, minority women of lower socioeconomic status and educational levels. The samples in the two large-sample clinic-based studies presented at the workshop, while not nationally representative, had socioeconomic profiles similar to that found in the NSFG.†

Norplant use was also importantly affected by geography. Norplant users are less likely to reside in areas defined by the NSFG as rural, and use of the implant in 1995 was substantially lower in the northeastern portion of the United States than in the midwestern, southern, and western regions of the country, with the western region showing the highest utilization percentages. These regional differences were thought to be related to variations in service provision and were noted to be a matter requiring exploration.

---

*See Appendix A, *Presentation 7* (Darroch).

†See Appendix A, *Presentations 8* and *9,* hereafter "the Columbia study" and "the RTI/Emory/CMC study," respectively.

Workshop participants further noted that these patterns of Norplant adoption, together with the contextual data provided by the clinic-based studies, suggest that younger women are using Norplant primarily for birth spacing, while older women of higher parity, more likely to have been enrolled postpartum and less likely to want more children, are adopting Norplant as a long-term reversible alternative to tubal ligation. The observation was made that these pictures of method utilization point to two different market niches for Norplant: a larger group of younger women relatively early in their childbearing careers, attracted by the method's efficacy and convenience and using it for shorter-term spacing, and a smaller group of older women committed to wider spacing or possible termination of fertility but unsure about sterilization.

Method Continuation and Discontinuation

In addition to pregnancy rates, Table 2-1 summarized the Norplant continuation rates from 14 countries and, for three of those countries, continuation rates for the LNG ROD. First-year continuation rates were high for all countries, ranging from 76.0 in Scandinavian countries to 97.6 in Thailand. For those studies where 5-year continuation rates were available, the low was 25.0 percent in the Dominican Republic, the high Indonesia's 90.0 and 78.2 percent (in two studies), the next highest China's 72.1 percent.

What is missing from these figures is information about motivation. Until the sort of information from longitudinal, large-sample, clinic-based studies such as those reported on at the workshop became available, understanding of the causes of method continuation and discontinuation was limited. Several workshop participants commented, however, that these studies were not fully representative. For instance, clinics already experienced with Norplant had been chosen for Postmarketing Surveillance because they had the infrastructure, research experience, and managerial capabilities to conduct the necessary epidemiological follow-up at an appropriate level of quality. Good service conditions, careful counseling, and meticulous follow-up would be expected in such settings and would also be expected to contribute to high continuation rates. Similar comments were made concerning the Columbia and RTI/Emory/CMC studies, which had been located in sites with what could be deemed model programs. The response was that the sites were not selected for that reason but because their programs were large enough to provide good-size samples, as well as to enable investigators to examine issues of "steering" onto Norplant and barriers to removal, assumed to be more likely among the poor minority women who were the principal clientele of the study clinics.

Nonetheless, there was agreement that, regardless of possible bias, clinic-based studies of this type, especially those with large samples, remain valuable. They are especially useful because the NSFG and the 1996 Ortho Birth Control Study had found too few Norplant users to permit extensive analysis and because clinics are generally so important in the provision of contraceptives. According to preliminary NSFG data reported at the workshop, of women using reversible contraceptives in 1995, 34 percent had obtained them from a clinic. Several presenters further observed that more broadly based studies, in other industrialized countries, in facilities with different client profiles, and in other delivery modalities (e.g., a sample of managed care facilities), would be highly desirable, crucial if implants of shorter terms of efficacy are to enter the market as options for a broader user population.

Table 2-2 displays continuation rates found in the studies presented at the workshop and from three additional study analyses provided for comparative purposes; it also includes information on the primary factors associated with continuation and discontinuation. The table shows that continuation rates at one year did not fall below 71 percent for any of these samples, a critical time marker since menstrual problems tend to have settled down for many women at the same time that discontinuation to start another pregnancy has not yet become a dominant factor. By the end of Norplant's approved 5-year term of use, approximately one-half of the users in these samples were continuing with the method. Although there are great differences by country and although the data for the United States are scanty (partly because of low utilization), Norplant continuation rates are high even at the 5-year mark. And, while explicitly comparative data are also scanty, continuation rates for the implant are high compared to those for other reversible methods.

Side Effects as Factors

Side effects have been generally considered major contributors to Norplant discontinuation, so that it was not surprising that the women in the Columbia and RTI/Emory/CMC studies said that what they liked least about Norplant were its side effects. As indicated above, because Norplant contains no estrogen, the most frequent side effects are changes in menstrual patterns, predominantly prolonged or irregular menstrual flow or increased bleeding. The general pattern is that the number of bleeding plus spotting days tends to be high during the first 6 to 9 months of use, stabilizing by the end of the first year at some level that becomes acceptable to a majority of continuing users. Overall, it is these effects that appear with the greatest frequency in all samples studied, including the large-sample Postmarketing Surveillance and Population Council studies discussed earlier. In the Population Council studies, menstrual problems in themselves accounted for discontinuation in the same proportions as all other side effects combined, at both 1 year and 5 years of use. Among those side effects, headache, vaginal discharge, pelvic pain, weight gain, and acne were the most frequent contributors.

The findings from the Columbia and RTI/Emory/CMC studies suggest that the role of side effects in decisions to continue or discontinue implant use may not always be clear-cut. As a general matter, there are variabilities in reported frequencies of side effects from sample to sample, from time point to time point, and in priority. There is also the question of whether a single side effect is determining or is part of a number of effects that prove determining in the aggregate. Some of the lack of clarity also derives from differences in terminology and analytic methodologies from study to study. Although menstrual changes[14] were, indeed, the most common reasons given for Norplant discontinuation at 6 months post-insertion, the Columbia study found that both "continuers" and "discontinuers" reported menstrual side effects at virtually equivalent levels. The study analysis concluded that women continuing implant use at 6 months were prepared to tolerate menstrual side effects, while women discontinuing at that time were not. In contrast, the RTI/Emory/CMC study found that women with severe menstrual side effects were more likely to discontinue use. It would seem that, absent a fuller understanding of such qualitative aspects as perceived severity and the implications of menstrual side effects for individual women, those effects are, in themselves, unreliable predictors of "early" method discontinuation.

Both the Columbia and RTI/Emory/CMC studies also found differences between continuers and discontinuers with respect to *nonmenstrual* side effects. In the Columbia sample, women who opted for discontinuation at 6 months were more likely to have experienced headaches, hair loss, and weight gain. In the RTI/Emory/CMC sample, at 12 months, while both menstrual and nonmenstrual side effects from Norplant each increased discontinuation, discontinuation attributed by women to nonmenstrual side effects was higher.

The RTI/Emory/CDC study examined the frequency of Norplant-related side effects relative to other contraceptive methods and found that nearly all Norplant users reported one or more side effects, as was the case for women using Depo-Provera; considerably fewer women using oral contraceptives (OCs) reported side effects. Norplant users experienced the largest number of side effects, more Norplant users defined their side effects as "severe" and, as shown below, more were somewhat less satisfied, yet their continuation rates were considerably higher than those for the other two methods.

Table 2-2 also shows that, in those studies that were designed to compare method use, implant continuation rates tend to be high relative to those of other reversible contraceptives. For example, in the Columbia sample, 50 percent of all women discontinuing use of Depo-Provera had done so after their first injection.

User Satisfaction

Data from the 1996 Ortho Birth Control study that were presented at the workshop in conjunction with the NSFG data showed favorable perceptions of Norplant tied with Depo-Provera at a 22 percent rating, ahead of the IUD's 15 percent but well behind tubal ligation, vasectomy, the male condom, and the pill (55, 63, 66, and 78 percent, respectively). The additional comment was made that preliminary indications from the NSFG data will also show that Depo-Provera is a less popular method than has been perceived by many providers who have tended to view it as more popular than Norplant.[15]

TABLE 2-2 Continuation Rates Among Implant[a] Users, Selected Pre- and Postmarketing Studies

Description, Sample (n/n)[b]	Continuing Use at: 1 Year	Continuing Use at: Later Study Years	Factors in Continuation	Factors in Discontinuation
Pre-introductory clinical trials in 17 countries; Population Council/FHI combined data set; 16,282 women aged 18–40, mean age 24–33, mean parity 1.8–5.8 births; follow-up at 1, 3, 6 mos. post-insertion, semi-annually or annually thereafter; 1984–1990.[c]	Highest: 97.0, Ghana, Philippines, Singapore Lowest: 71.1, Brazil	At 5 years, highest: 64.2 Lowest: 40.0, Bangladesh	No data	Younger age and higher parity at insertion were consistently associated with higher discontinuation rates after Year 1 for the whole data set. Menstrual problems were the chief reason for discontinuation in 6 countries; in 5 countries, desired pregnancy was the primary reason. Largest increases in cumulative discontinuation rates for desired pregnancy were in Years 4 and 5. Highest discontinuation rates for "other medical" reasons were found in Latin America in Years 1, 2, and 3.
Pre-introductory trial, San Francisco; 250 women, 70% with LNG ROD; 5 years; 1986–1989.[d]	No data	At 5 years: 46.0	Implant chosen because of prior problems with contraception, view that easy to use, belief in long efficacy.	Nonmenstrual side effects (mainly weight gain, acne) were the prime catalyst for discontinuation. Most users experienced at least one side effect: menstrual changes, 82%; weight changes, 32%; headaches, 24%; mood changes, 16%; and acne, 15%.

Study description		Findings
Prospective observational; convenience sample; inner-city clinic; 122 largely minority women aged 13–19, parity at least 1, most already clinic clients; structured interview plus chart review follow-up; 6/91–6/93.[e]	71.0 At 2 years: 62.0	Age, race, weight, parity, and school status were not predictive of retention. Past history of 1 or more induced abortions only statistically significant predictor distinguishing continuers and discontinuers.	After 6 months, social reasons (including desire for pregnancy) were the most common reasons for discontinuation, although sample had preselected only teens intending to delay pregnancy at least 3 years. "General symptoms" (headache, fatigue, hair loss, nausea, breast symptoms, weight changes, appetite changes) were frequently reported by discontinuers in first 6 months, rarely later. Menstrual irregularities were uncommon reasons for termination, especially after first 6 months.
Clinical trial, 600 women with LNG ROD, 598 with Norplant "soft tubing" implants, randomized sample, 7 clinics, 3 years. 6/90–2/94.[f]	93.0 At 3 years: 80.0	Women not indicating at outset that they wanted another pregnancy were significantly more likely to continue use. Continuation rates for women whose family was completed were over 90 per 100.	Menstrual problems (more bleeding days, irregular and/or increased bleeding) were associated with higher termination rate than were medical problems (headache, weight gain, acne), planning pregnancy, or other personal reasons.

Continued

TABLE 2-2 Continued

| | Continuing Use at: | | | |
Description, Sample (n/n)[b]	1 Year	Later Study Years	Factors in Continuation	Factors in Discontinuation
Postmarketing surveillance, 16,000 in eight countries, over 5 years.[g]	No data	67.0	Continuation at 5 years was equal to IUD (65%–66%). Careful selection of clients well motivated to use long-term reversible method.	>15% discontinued for medical reasons, notably bleeding irregularities (8% among IUD users).
Longitudinal 5-year study, 910/2,003 poor, mostly young minority women, urban hospital-based clinics (Dallas, New York, Pittsburgh); 5/93–10/96.[h]	77.0	2-year data not ready for publication	Continuation with Depo-Provera at 12 months post-initiation, 45%.	Prime predictors of "early" discontinuation were partner wanting child, dissatisfaction with prior contraceptive methods, and exposure to negative media coverage.
Longitudinal 4-year study; 2,477 young, mostly postpartum, poor minority women; urban (Charlotte, NC, Atlanta) family planning/postpartum clinics, maternity wards, ambulatory surgery: 7/93–10/94.[i]	86.0	2- and 3-year data not ready for publication	Continuation rates for both Depo-Provera and the pill at 12 months were considerably lower.	Rates of Norplant, pill, and Depo-Provera discontinuation were highest in women with menstrual side effects subjectively defined as "severe." More Norplant users had more side effects but even for those with "severe" side effects, 1-year discontinuation rate was lowest for implants. Pattern for nonmenstrual side effects was similar.

[a]The implant studied was Norplant® except where otherwise indicated.
[b]n/n = number of users evaluated out of number enrolled in study. Dates refer to enrollment period.

cGrubb GS, D Moore, NG Anderson, et al. Pre-introductory clinical trials of Norplant implants: A comparison of 17 countries' experience. *Contraception* 52:287–296, 1995. All the Norplant capsules in these studies were made with the "hard tubing" which releases slightly lower levels of steroid than the currently marketed capsules. The authors believe that the great disparities in adverse events data are artifactual, probably resulting from differences in reporting practices.

dDarney PD, E Atkinson, S Tanner, S MacPherson, et al. Acceptance and perceptions of Norplant® among users in San Francisco, USA. *Studies in Family Planning* 21(3):152–160, 1990.

eSivin I, O Viegas, I Campodinico, et al. Clinical performance of a new two-rod levonorgestrel contraceptive implant: A 3-year randomized study with Norplant® implants as controls. *Contraception* 55:73–80, 1997. Clinics were in Bangkok, Chile (2), Finland, New York City, and Singapore.

fGlantz S, E Schaff, N Campbell-Heider, et al. Contraceptive implant use among inner-city teens. *Journal of Adolescent Health* 16:389–395, 1995.

gWHO/HRP, Population Council, Family Health International. Data from International Collaborative Postmarketing Surveillance, presented at Workshop on Implant Contraceptives, Washington, D.C., Institute of Medicine, 7–8 April 1997. (See *Presentation 1* [Meirik].)

hKalmuss D, and A Davidson. Norplant Discontinuation among Low-Income Women. Supported by the National Institute of Child Health and Human Development and the Henry J. Kaiser Family Foundation. Data presented at Workshop on Implant Contraceptives, Washington, D.C., Institute of Medicine, 7–8 April 1997. (See also *Presentation 8* [Kalmuss, Davidson]—Davidson A, D Kalmuss, L Cushman, S Heartwell, and M Rulin. Determinants of early implant discontinuation among 166 low-income women. *Family Planning Perspectives* 28(6):256–260, 1996; Davidson A, D Kalmuss, L Cushman, D Romero, S Heartwell, and M Rulin. Injectable contraceptive discontinuation and subsequent unintended pregnancy among low-income women. *American Journal of Public Health* 87:1532–1534, 1997.)

iKoo HP, JD Griffith, ME Nennstiel, WL Graves, RA Hatcher, and S Laurent. Women's Experience with Norplant: A Comparison with Depo-Provera and Oral Contraceptives. Research Triangle Institute, Emory University, and Carolinas Medical Center. Supported by the National Institute of Child Health and Human Development and the Henry J. Kaiser Family Foundation. Data presented at Workshop on Implant Contraceptives, Washington, D.C., Institute of Medicine, 7–8 April 1997. (See *Presentation 9* [Koo].)

The RTI/Emory/CMC study found that the majority[16] of the women who continued Norplant use were "very satisfied" with the method, while noting that they had not found it easy to get used to. While that satisfaction level was below the satisfaction levels for Depo-Provera and OCs, nearly all Norplant continuers would recommend the method to others; not as many would do so, however, for each of the other two methods. Not surprisingly, perceptions among those discontinuing Norplant use were reported as less positive: Very few indicated that they had been very satisfied, compared to sizable minorities of those who had discontinued use of Depo-Provera and oral contraceptives. Whether they continued or discontinued Norplant use, both groups perceived that the best features of Norplant were its convenience and effectiveness; fewer Depo-Provera and OC users, whether continuers or discontinuers, cited those attributes as "their" method's best features.

The workshop presentations and discussion concluded that much remains to be understood before anyone can make broad assertions about reasons for continuing and discontinuing use of the contraceptive implant and about how those reasons differ from population to population over the reproductive cycle. Menstrual disturbances and other medical reasons are undeniably important but, overall, reasons for retaining or removing Norplant are a complex blend of personal experience of side effects, "other-directed" variables like the wishes of partners and broader social influences, the passage of time, and changes in life plans. Several participants commented that what seems to be happening is that women who stay with Norplant seem motivated to trade off side effects, even when burdensome in number or severity, for the convenience and efficacy they believe essential to greater control over their lives.

Barriers to Discontinuation

Norplant continuation rates may be high relative to other methods simply because a surgical intervention is required for discontinuation, unlike Depo-Provera and the pill which users can stop of their own accord. A related point is that women who must first surmount the mental barrier of deciding to experience another surgical procedure, albeit minor, then may face either real or anticipated barriers in the form of clinical pressure for continuation and/or financial costs associated with removal.

These issues were examined in both the Columbia and RTI/Emory/CMC studies, which looked at the two primary points at which pressure might be placed on women at the provider level: the point of initial method election and the point of deciding to discontinue method use—that is, removal. In terms of the first potential pressure point, the Columbia study found that of the 2,000 women interviewed, only three reported feeling pressure from a health care provider to use Norplant. Choice had instead been predicated on perceived convenience, effectiveness, and duration; in fact, Norplant electors found the method more difficult to obtain than oral contraceptives.

The second potential pressure point examined was whether provider- or cost-based barriers impeded access to Norplant removal. Here, presenters noted a mixed picture. The finding in the RTI/Emory/CMC study was that slightly over 15 percent of the women in that sample who planned, considered, or actually proceeded to remove Norplant had perceived provider pressure not to do so; in addition, those women had to pay more visits to the clinic to obtain removal and expressed considerably less satisfaction with these clinic visits. Preliminary evidence from the Columbia study indicated that for some women, cost factors did act as an impediment to Norplant removal. While the great majority of women did not perceive that cost factors would make it more difficult to obtain implant removal, those who did were significantly less likely to discontinue Norplant use.

In summary, although the great preponderance of women, at least in these clinic settings, did not encounter barriers to removal, workshop participants agreed that the fact problems were encountered points to the need for improvements in clinic policy and in provider education in several areas. The most critical of those are method costs and financing, assurance of removal, and how to communicate this information to women clearly and effectively—needs pertinent, in fact, to any long-acting, provider-dependent contraceptive method. None of these are small challenges, participants observed. The price of Norplant remains an issue and providers have a delicate balance to strike between helping women tolerate side effects without conveying the sense that removal is being resisted for any reason.

Cost and Cost-Effectiveness

In its *Contraceptive Research and Development* report, the 1996 committee argued that contraception was highly cost-effective and recommended continued and sufficient government support of contraceptive services and the inclusion by third-party payers of contraception as a covered service, particularly for low-income individuals and in developing countries.[17] In this connection, the committee believed that examination of experience with Norplant would usefully include consideration of its cost-effectiveness.

*Presentation 10** began with the premise that at the core of contraceptive cost and effectiveness is the relationship among initial method cost, duration of use, and pregnancies averted. A "savings" model was developed for the United States that calculated a total cost for each of 15 categories of reversible and irreversible contraceptives and the costs of pregnancies resulting from contraceptive failure based on the four possible unintended pregnancy outcomes—spontaneous abortion, ectopic pregnancy, induced abortion, or birth—each in the proportion expected nationally in the United States. All costs were derived from a state Medicaid schedule of benefits and compared to a private payer database. The model also incorporated assumptions about time horizons, since some contraceptive methods require a greater one-time (e.g., sterilization) or initial (e.g.,

---

*See Appendix A, *Presentation 10* (Stewart).

implant) investment which would bias a 1-year time frame considerably. Periods of use of 1 through 5 years were calculated for all methods, together with their cumulative costs over 5 years, to locate the point at which investment in a given method would become cost-effective compared to use of no method or compared to all other methods.

The analysis made it clear that all forms of contraception, including dual-method use, are far less costly in the United States than an unintended pregnancy. In the array of individual method costs and associated savings, whose rank order is driven largely by their relative failure rates, by their consequences in the form of unintended pregnancy, and by the high price of pregnancy, the implant ranks very high in cost-effectiveness relative to other contraceptive methods, saving $13,813 over a 5-year period of use. This is the case even for younger users, for whom a pregnancy prevented is typically delayed rather than averted (in which instance savings are reduced), and even though the method entails substantial initial costs.[18]

However, while amortization of costs over time may make sense for planners, the subcommittee's analysis was that it is far less meaningful for the user who needs to find the total funds up front, as well as for providers subsidizing that up-front payment. Because it has not been possible to negotiate a public-sector price for Norplant, its cost was an issue for U.S. public-sector (Title X) clinics which are generally affected by repeated struggles for reasonable levels of program funding. In the case of Norplant, some of those clinics found themselves dependent on financial help from foundations for keeping adequate quantities of the method on their shelves. Ironically, such clinics, as a group, may have inserted more implants and, some participants commented, done the best screening and counseling in the nation.

Participants also raised the question of what happens to amortization of costs when users discontinue use of a long-term contraceptive method prior to termination of its full term of approved use, 5 years in the case of Norplant. They noted the tension this establishes—citing examples from publicly funded or managed care contexts, in the United States and in at least one developing country (Indonesia)—in terms of provider and client concerns about the size of the initial investment in Norplant insertion and the corresponding loss when use is discontinued. To these may be added concerns about additional costs—either to provider or client—associated with removal earlier than might have been hoped or expected. In some settings, these concerns have been expressed as pressure (anticipated or expressed) on women not to have the implant removed. Yet another source of tension in some program settings is the fact that while implant insertion is free of cost to the client, removal is not.

Furthermore, because Norplant's approved term of efficacy is 5 years, there has been a tendency to view it as a method *intended* for a 5-year period of use, not as a method that *can provide* effective contraception for *up to* 5 years.[19] This perception has prompted such concepts as "early" or "premature" removal, and an emphasis on 5-year continuation rates as critical indicators of the acceptability of and satisfaction with the method. Thus, method "switching" may be affected by concerns among some users and providers about costs. This fits poorly with the fact that freedom to change methods is generally considered a good thing in family planning, as well as with the fact that many women may want to use Norplant to space births at intervals considerably shorter than 5 years.

Data from the RTI/Emory/CMC studies suggest that women who discontinue Norplant use seem much less likely than women who discontinue use of the pill or Depo-Provera to switch to exposed non-use, and much more likely to switch to an effective contraceptive method. In that case, the costs of unintended pregnancy that act as the main driver in the savings model would be attenuated. These conclusions were based on a small sample and may be too subtle for a standard cost-effectiveness analysis; they do point to the vulnerability of cost-effectiveness arguments to circumstances and to the vagaries of human behavior.

Effects of Media Coverage and Litigation on Norplant Use

A point of debate at the workshop had to do with what constituted the precipitating event in the sudden decline in Norplant utilization in the United States that began in early 1994.[*] Some participants thought that communication among individual users about their negative experiences with the method had been the primary stimulus; others thought that it had been media coverage; others thought it was the litigation itself. Figure 2-1 is an attempt to sort out these differing perceptions by tracking patterns of Norplant insertions, women's opinions about the method, events in the courts, and media coverage.

The figure shows coincidence among decline in method adoption, negative attitudes, legal actions, and media coverage of those actions. While previous years had shown periods of decline in Norplant adoption, there had been a regular rhythm to those declines at the end of each calendar year that was interpreted as a general seasonal falloff in family planning clinic attendance. The pattern for 1994 was, however, distinctive. The sequence displayed in the figure would suggest that the catalytic event was arguably the March 1994 suit filed by Chicago lawyer Jewel Klein, followed by the first broad public airing in May 1994 of the fact that some women were undergoing difficult implant removals. This does not exclude—and may even imply—an effect from communication among individual users; however, that dynamic might have remained a largely local phenomenon had conversations about Norplant not become a matter for the media. Media coverage of method problems expanded from that point, negative attitudes toward Norplant mounted, and the number of adoptions fell in a straight-line pattern unlike the patterns of the preceding 2 years.

The Columbia study, which had begun to gather data in spring 1993, was expanded in August 1994 to incorporate questions concerning the effect of these dynamics on women's decisions about method adoption and continuation. Preliminary analysis of those data indicates that the large majority of the total study sample reported exposure to media coverage of Norplant-related events; of these, a similarly large majority had heard negative coverage, and a significant

---

[*]The reader is also referred to the chronological material in Appendix B.

minority of the "media-exposed" women had been motivated to seek removal by what they had gathered from various media sources. The RTI/Emory/CMC study, which began in July 1993, encountered a sharp decline in the proportion of women choosing Norplant in the third quarter (July–September) of 1994. This decline was attributed to a decrease in that quarter in the proportion of women who thought that the method was "very effective" or "very convenient," or who were favorably disposed toward using it.

Other pertinent data come from the Ortho Birth Control Survey, data that could not, for mechanical reasons, be well reflected in Figure 2-1. In 1994, of the Ortho sample of women aged 15–50, 34 percent had had a favorable opinion of Norplant, with 16 percent viewing it unfavorably. By 1995, these percentages had shifted to 22 percent and 38 percent, respectively, with the better than doubling in unfavorable views coming from those women in the previous year's sample who had had no opinion.

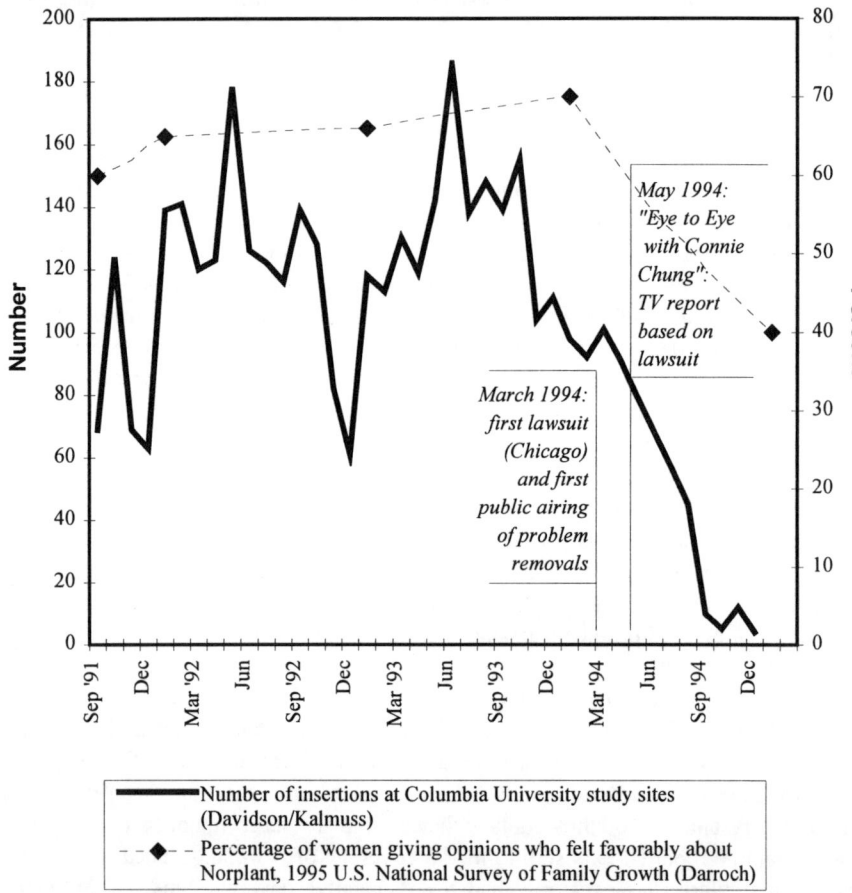

FIGURE 2-1. Implant insertions, women's opinions about Norplant, and key events. SOURCES: *Presentations 7* (Darroch) and *8* (Davidson/Kalmuss) and staff research.

INSERTION AND REMOVAL: EXPERIENCE AND IMPLICATIONS

This series of presentations addressed the technical elements of implant insertion and, most particularly, removal,[*] and the demands those placed on the introduction of Norplant into the United Kingdom,[†] the United States,[‡] and Indonesia.[§]

Technical Aspects

A distinguishing feature of Norplant is the requirement that a provider insert and remove it. Though both insertion and removal may seem simple procedures, for virtually all providers there are two learning curves: one associated with putting the device in, the other with taking it out. Done correctly, a proper insertion allows a provider to feel the capsules in a fan-like arrangement beneath the skin. These are the easiest removals. However, when the insertion is poorly done, the capsules may be in uneven relationships with one another. This is generally not a problem while the implant remains *in situ* but it may well produce complications when a provider, often not the same individual who inserted it, attempts removal.

Three removal methods currently predominate: (1) the "standard" method, used in Norplant introductory training in the United States; (2) the "pop-out" method, requiring more precision and, some said, more time; and, (3) the "U" technique, which removes the implanted capsules in a U-shaped fashion. For all methods, removal proceeds following injection with a local anesthetic near the base of the fan of capsules. The U technique, developed and evaluated in Indonesia as a possible alternative method, was described as requiring less manual dexterity than the other two methods, as well as less training time for acquisition of sustained competency; it also was reported to produce fewer removal problems and shorter removal times.

Case Experiences

Introduction of Norplant into the United Kingdom was based on pre-introductory market research among providers and consumers by the method's distributor, Hoechst Marion Roussel, research that provided early understanding about what was most likely to make Norplant's introduction as problem-free as possible. The findings were that success would depend on high awareness about the implant among clinicians (known to be unenthusiastic about progestin-only

---

[*] See Appendix A, *Presentation 11* (Archer).
[†] See Appendix A, *Presentation 12* (Davey and Gaffikin).
[‡] See Appendix A, *Presentation 13* (Blumenthal).
[§] See Appendix A, *Presentation 14* (Simmons).

methods), on documented competency, on appropriate client selection and fully informative counseling, and on generous training support and follow-up. Another and very crucial element of success would be training not only for insertion but for removal because, beyond the progestin-related side effects of the implant's contents, the program designers anticipated that implant removal would be a significant issue. The program first trained a small core group of senior trainers on site in Indonesia and then used them to precipitate a "cascade" of training and one-on-one supervised clinical practice for selected providers in 35 training centers nationwide. A checklist was developed to standardize the stages to competency in training for both insertions and removals.

In the United States, the training process was different. Before putting Norplant on the U.S. market, its distributor, Wyeth-Ayerst, provided support for a national hands-on training program in Norplant insertion for physicians, nurse practitioners, and physicians' assistants, using master trainers in 37 hospital- and clinic-based locations. However, the master trainers did not constitute a standing corps as was the case in the United Kingdom, making consistency a problem. Furthermore, for the most part, it had to be left to individual practitioners to present themselves for training, and this did not always happen. A number of participants expressed the opinion that the apparent simplicity of the procedure and general optimism about the technology blocked recognition that insertion and removal each required different learning curves and that successful removals would depend greatly on proper insertion. The observation was also made that there had been little anticipation that removals would, in fact, be a major issue, at least in the foreseeable future.

In Indonesia,[20] the major issues in training, especially for removal, emerged when the program went from field trials in three provinces to full-scale nationwide introduction. Implant removal on demand had been assured during trials and program managers had welcomed the need for training in removal techniques. The new method was initially popular and had potential for expanding a range of contraceptive choice that was limited by cultural sanctions on sterilization. However, when the method went to scale, provider attitudes described by evaluators as "authoritarian," lack of time for adequate counseling, and community pressures meant that women often got the message that they were making a 5-year commitment; later, those who sought removal before 5 years encountered resistance. And, though program managers recognized that not enough providers had been appropriately trained in removal skills, they felt that they had 5 years to catch up in this regard. However, at the end of that period, the volume of need, time pressures, logistical problems, and lack of resources highlighted the reality that catch-up had not, in fact, occurred and that many providers had been inadequately prepared in both insertion and removal techniques. The result was a backlog of from 350,000 to 500,000 implants awaiting removal. The weight of the lessons learned from this experience was sufficient to prompt WHO/HRP to seek fresh strategies for introducing new contraceptives, described below in the section on "New Approaches."

Rates of Complicated Removals

The rate of removal difficulties reported from Postmarketing Surveillance was 1 percent. Of 7,977 Norplant insertions, 4 were problematic and, of the 7,827 removals that had occurred by 5 years of use, 79 had been difficult, 46 of those in the same two clinics. The rate in the Population Council studies was 2.6 percent for both Norplant and the LNG ROD. Both rates are low compared to the removal complication rate of 6.2 percent in clinical trials that appears in the product labeling.[21] As some workshop participants noted, the Surveillance studies and the non-randomized Population Council studies were conducted in family planning clinics chosen for their good quality, all of which had had experience with Norplant and were familiar with both insertion and removal procedures.

The workshop accounts and ancillary material provided by presenters indicated that approximately 95 percent of removals were successful without significant problems. At the same time, some workshop participants thought that the fact that removal problems were lower in clinics chosen as research sites suggested that the 5 to 7 percent of removals that were problematic were largely avoidable and could be preemptively addressed in the future; others thought that these were probably optimal situations.

Implications

As noted in the preceding section, implant removal was the catalyst for what quickly became a critical mass of opinion and events that led to the decline in Norplant use not just in the United States but, as the presenter from the United Kingdom observed, in that country as well. The core issues were provider training and competency in implant insertion and removal, real or imputed coercion of users not to remove the implant, and the character of counseling about method use in general. Workshop participants concurred that deficits in each of these had contributed, in different degrees, to litigation, negative media coverage, and loss of confidence in the method among providers and consumers.

The subcommittee diagnosis of the complexities of training for Norplant had several parts. The first had to do with the fact that introduction of new medical technologies typically requires education in their use. While many new medical devices and surgical techniques are introduced gradually, often through academic medical centers, this was not so with Norplant. The implant system was introduced countrywide and its initial market penetration grew so rapidly that the base of deliverers, though broad, was not deep; this was the case in the United States as well as in the very large Indonesian program. The combination of speed and lack of depth proved to be especially problematic when removals subsequently became an issue.

Discussion during the workshop and the subcommittee's executive session advanced the notion that medical culture and attitudes had also contributed to training problems. Many physicians apparently felt that this new, simple technology did not require special training and they therefore were not motivated to find time in inevitably demanding schedules for training. An analysis of the training experience presented at the workshop made the point that medical training, undergraduate or postgraduate, is often provided in circumstances where competency is not demonstrated, documented, or required before use.[22] The presentation noted that in one limited assessment, a physician's assistant who had undergone formal training in implant removal and for whom it became a regular procedure demonstrated faster removal times and fewer problems than a physician who was largely self-taught.[23]

The second explanation considered by the subcommittee had to do with another general question in medicine: Who is the first patient for any invasive procedure? When the implant was being introduced in the United States, there were relatively small numbers of users and therefore an even smaller number of women requesting removal. As a consequence, training was predominantly limited to a model arm. Recent analysis (not reported at the workshop) indicates that even with ideal placement, practitioners may require at least five trials to become proficient in removal.[24] Thousands of women thus became "first patients" for Norplant insertions and, later, removals, and there were reports to the effect that women did not always understand that they were, in effect, participating in a training program, particularly in situations where language and social distance were issues. The subcommittee marked this as a chronic dilemma in medical practice, partly resolved by the manual dexterity the clinician has already accumulated that could be applied to new procedures, partly by informing patients that trainees are involved in performing that procedure, and partly by good supervision.

A third set of issues related to the fact that, despite earnest efforts, training in the insertion and removal of Norplant was uneven, most acutely with respect to removal, an unevenness deriving largely from the health care system structures into which the method was introduced. The presentation on the experience in the United Kingdom made the point that the organization of the national health system made it possible to develop and implement a standardized training program tailored to the needs of family practitioners, who provide 80 percent of contraception as a regular part of the comprehensive care of their patients. In contrast, the U.S. system did not lend itself easily or rapidly to uniformity of medical education or practice. As observed earlier, while one-third of the Norplant users identified by the NSFG obtained the method through family planning clinics, two-thirds obtained it from a miscellany of sources. In neither country is there a legal way to prevent any physician who wishes to do so from inserting or removing the implant.

Where training environments were created in which practitioners had to prove competency before training in the patient setting, and where standardized checklists were developed for proficiency and prediction of difficult removals, procedure times fell and patient satisfaction rose. This, with the experience in the United Kingdom, was seen by workshop participants as evidence that client attitudes about Norplant can be altered by provision of safe and expedient removal. Participants commented that new removal techniques and the greater simplicity of the LNG ROD described by workshop presenters should be helpful, especially if those techniques are somehow standardized. However, they added, the need for appropriate training—in insertion, removal, and communication with clients—persists.

CONSUMER PERSPECTIVES[*]

This section presents the main themes that emerged from a dialogue led by a panel that assembled perspectives from women's health advocacy, reproductive ethics, and the clinic. While no such panel could be fully representative, in combination with the other constituencies represented at the workshop it encompassed a fair range of experience and opinion. The intent was to capture aspects of the Norplant experience that evade statistics and to further a dialogue that, some participants noted, should have begun years ago. The observation was made that the power of perceptions in the history of contraceptive technology has been great, even when dismissed as unsubstantial or too anecdotal to be considered "real" data.

The issues raised in what became extensive discussion fall into three related categories of concern: (1) communication and quality of care, (2) informed decision-making, and, (3) consumer involvement. A fourth category—cultural, sociopolitical, and socioeconomic factors—was woven through the others.

Communication and Quality of Care

The importance of information, education, and communication—"I, E, and C"—has been a theme in family planning for years, so it was not surprising to hear it cited as critical in Norplant's history. Taking the material presented at the workshop, as well as their own experiences, as their point of departure, the panelists constructed a picture of what counseling and communication should be, with respect to Norplant and to long-acting contraceptives in general. The panelists described a continuum that would span

- appropriate and intelligible product labeling, and
- provider training, including

    — collaboration in initial method choice,

---

[*]This section summarizes perspectives presented by Katz, Macklin, Moskowitz, Pearson, Scott, and Secundy, interwoven with perspectives from the workshop group as a whole.

— support for clients in dealing with side effects, possible discontinuation, and removal on demand or as approved efficacy ends and a new contraceptive choice must be made.

Counseling would optimally occur as truly two-way dialogue in which:

- information exchanged and necessary understandings are complete and unconstrained by time,
- client participation in contraceptive choice is truly voluntary, and
- hierarchical distinctions between provider and client are muted to the extent necessary for all this to happen.

Quality of Care

The panelists described what the policy and institutional support for this communication continuum would look like in the case of contraceptive implants. That support would include

- assurance of choice,
- removal on demand,
- final removal on time, and
- capacity for following clients through each of these segments of need.

They added that the medical system's role in sustaining contraception—that is, helping women stay on a method yet change freely as appropriate—would, ideally, integrate contraceptive counseling into reproductive health care, including sexual health, and more broadly into comprehensive medical care. For both Norplant and the LNG ROD, this entails special attention during the first 6 to 9 months when bleeding patterns are most irregular, as well as thoughtful, open response if removal becomes necessary. The panelists concurred in the impression that where these characteristics had prevailed, Norplant continuation was high; where they did not, continuation rates were lower and, in some cases, problems ensued. One participant remarked that as the most complex contraceptive ever introduced onto the market, Norplant had placed sizable demands on even the best clinical situations.

Informed Decision-Making

Presenters and participants returned throughout the workshop to the following issues: (1) the importance of informed decision-making; (2) the nature and adequacy of the content of the information provided in clinical settings; (3) the special challenges of long-acting contraceptives; and, (4) community involvement in preparing for introduction of new contraceptive methods, especially methods that history suggests might lend themselves to abuse.

Importance

Use of the terms "informed decision-making" and "informed choice" are increasingly recognized as desirable since they clearly convey the importance of informing for purposes of dissent as well as consent. These terms and the issues around them were flagged as especially crucial for groups of lower socioeconomic status, in developing and developed countries.

Content

For Norplant, an informed decision-making process would entail discussion of:

- the removal option and cost implications;
- other method options;
- relative risks, benefits, and discomforts associated with each option; and
- the need for additional protection from sexually transmitted disease.

Participants also noted the need for ongoing review—by manufacturers, providers, and system managers—to ensure that information critical to method choice is provided in appropriate formats. The discussion centered on how to adapt such information to account for differences in educational levels, language, socioeconomic status, and stage of the reproductive life span, and on the need for innovative methodologies such as modern commercial marketing techniques and focus-group approaches to accomplish this.

Special Challenges

The crux of the discussion of informed decision-making was that long-acting contraceptives that depend on a clinical provider for discontinuation (implants, IUD) or require users to wait until contraceptive effect wears off (Depo-Provera) also require management strategies different from reversible methods that can be stopped at the will of the user. The sense of some advocacy representatives is that provider dependence requires a routine policy that adopters record their understanding of, and acquiescence to, the necessary procedures through formal mechanisms usually referred to as "informed consent" documents. The rationale is that even if such instruments dissuade some prospective users, fewer "happier" users are—and, they argued, would have been in the case of Norplant—a net good. Some participants called attention to the constraints imposed by such procedures on access to contraceptives, and to such generic dilemmas as intelligibility and differences in the nature of consent in clinical research and in actual product use. Still, there was a strong sense among the panelists and most participants that in the case of contraceptives, more information is preferable to less; again, fewer more but well-informed contraceptive users were viewed as preferable to more but poorly informed ones.

Potential for Abuse

There was much discussion of legislative and judicial attempts in the United States beginning in 1991 to utilize Norplant coercively: by mandating its use as a condition of probation in cases of child abuse, making it a precondition for access to welfare payments, or offering financial incentives to welfare recipients to adopt it.[25] None of these efforts succeeded. However, because they had focused primarily on poor, single women, often black or Hispanic, they had evoked memories of other, previous attempts to restrict reproductive freedom[26] that had disproportionately affected minority women. This added to an existing residue of suspicion in some quarters,[27] affected objective assessment of the method itself, and highlighted the need for special regard to ensure reproductive choice in the provision of long-acting, provider-dependent contraceptive methods as a general matter. Reports indicated that lack of free choice, in method election and continuation, had on occasion been an issue in some developing countries.

During these exchanges, several avenues of exploration were suggested for improving informed decision-making processes:

• development of core guidelines for introducing long-acting contraceptives and support for modifying those, as desired and suitable, in communities where there have been attempts to use long-acting contraceptives inappropriately or where educational level, language, culture, or socioeconomic status may act as barriers to informed decision-making;

• participation of representatives from relevant groups in such communities in, first, developing procedures for informed decision-making that are understandable and truly informative and, second, crafting innovative communication modalities for achieving that goal; and

• more concrete, systematic training of providers in informed decision-making as an ongoing process that would include initial discussion about removal and ongoing discussion as needed, including help with the delicate distinctions between the provider's professional tendency to recommend the technological best for a patient and what might be interpreted as pressure.

The participants as a group recognized the complexities, subtleties, and practical challenges of pursuing these suggestions and acknowledged that doing so would require creativity, diligence, time, and expense, all of which challenge any clinical environment. They noted the additional difficulties when provider incentives run explicitly counter to free exercise of contraceptive choice. For example, when the Indonesian Norplant program went to scale, field staff were rewarded for numbers of adopters recruited, which fostered pressures on women to adopt. In the United Kingdom, the incentives were, and continue to be, in the other direction: Providers get a fee for IUD insertion but not for insertion of Norplant.

Consumer Involvement

In some countries, notably including the United States, opinions of policy makers and women's groups have diverged on a number of critical issues related to contraceptive research and development. These differences are significant because they have provoked domestic and international debates and controversies that have contributed to the persistent volatility in the contraceptives market.

The subcommittee's perception is that this has been changing for several reasons. One was the sponsorship beginning in 1991 by the WHO/HRP of meetings whose purpose was to bring women's health advocates and scientists to some kind of common ground. Another was the process of articulating the Program of Action of the 1994 United Nations International Conference on Population and Development (ICPD), which gave voice to a constituency for new types of partnerships between the public and private sectors, including women's and consumer groups, that would mobilize the experience and resources of industry while protecting the public interest. Yet another was the awareness, growing out of cumulative experience with the introduction of new contraceptives, that more care and creativity are needed. The revised perspective is that consumer involvement from the very outset should be integral to assessment of product need, iterative throughout all stages of product trial, and pivotal in product introduction and postmarketing surveillance.

NEW APPROACHES

The last set of workshop presentations described new approaches in key areas where answers are being sought to some of the problems that have contributed to the deficits in the current array of contraceptive options. Each approach takes on a different area of concern and each is described in the next section of this report. A very new activity, the "Boom and Bust Initiative," addresses the historically inadequate incorporation of consumer interests and concerns in all phases of the development, introduction, and use of contraceptive technologies. The WHO strategy approaches the full range of health system constraints to appropriate introduction and delivery of contraceptives. The Government Standards Defense offers a possible mechanism for dealing with the pressures of product liability on innovation in contraceptive research and development.

Reproductive Health Technologies Project's "Boom and Bust Initiative"

This presentation first described the Reproductive Health Technologies Project, the institutional home for this very new initiative. The Project, located in Washington, D.C., was founded in 1988 as a working group to provide public education in the United States about RU 486 and other antiprogestins. It subsequently expanded its scope and was established as a nonprofit organization in 1992. Today the Project brings together leaders from a wide range of constituencies and disciplines for dialogue, debate, and consensus-building on issues of reproductive health and technology, especially on highly charged issues where science, politics, and the interests of women converge and often clash.

The "Boom and Bust Initiative" was conceived as a response to concerns about what is now seen as a pattern of repeated difficulties when new contraceptive products are developed and introduced to consumers. The pattern described in this presentation is cyclical: high sales, demand, and expectations upon introduction of a new contraceptive method, followed by market collapse when the product does not fulfill all expectations or its use is inappropriate. Both parts of the cycle have obstructed realistic, nuanced, data-based understanding of product strengths and limitations, and the costs are high: diminished contraceptive choices; health problems for women using products inappropriately; negative impact on the financial well-being of companies; discouraged investment in contraceptive research and development; and a climate of mistrust and lack of confidence about the introduction and delivery of new contraceptive products which affects researchers, providers, and consumers.

The Initiative's goal is to engage key players—sometimes adversaries—in this cycle, in collaborative efforts to interrupt it.[28] The basic belief is that shared interest in meeting the contraceptive and reproductive health needs of consumers can motivate a diverse group to action, despite divergent views. The methodology will be a series of explorations of different perceptions of the cycle through case studies and carefully facilitated discussions. Possible outcomes include better working relationships among constituency groups, a "peace accord" outlining areas of agreement and future actions to which participants commit so as to avoid or disrupt the "Boom and Bust" cycle, and a monograph or documentary film chronicling the process and recounting points of consensus. The Initiative's objectives are not to achieve perfect consensus or collective will. Rather, they are, first, to understand past cycles so as to have the earliest possible input into the evolution of new contraceptives and, second, to constructively anticipate "break points" in their introduction.

The WHO Strategic Approach to Contraceptive Introduction

This presentation described a new endeavor on the part of WHO's Human Reproduction Program, based on analysis of experience with the introduction of new contraceptives in developing countries. Scrutiny of that experience revealed that simply making new contraceptives available does not necessarily expand either choice or utilization when basic constraints on delivering adequate services and responding to technical needs have not been addressed. Case studies have made it clear that failure has come from neglect of social and operational contexts. The elements of those contexts that were found to matter most were: inadequate preparation for introduction overall and, more specifically, inappropriate technical competence and counseling and inadequate logistics and supplies, support for the experience of side effects, assurance of method choice, provision of discontinuation on demand, and ability and willingness to support the additional program costs required to remedy all the above.

Recognition of these realities led WHO to broaden its framework for introduction from what was termed a "decontextualized" focus on single technologies to a focus that, in contrast, would take context very much into account. This would include what needed to be known about services and users in order to better inform policy decisions on method selection. The new approach emphasizes:

- method mix and reproductive choice;
- user perspectives and needs;
- service capacity for assuring voluntarism, quality of care, and affordable cost; and
- a participatory, multidisciplinary, "country-owned" process that promotes collaboration among governments, women's health and community groups, non-governmental providers, researchers, international donors, and technical assistance agencies.

The strategy proceeds in three stages:

- assessment of need for contraceptive introduction,
- research to inform decision-making on technology introduction and reproductive choice, and
- utilization of research for policy and planning.

Implementation is in different early stages in eight countries in four geographic regions.[29] All needs assessments have discovered major philosophical, structural, and managerial barriers to quality of care in reproductive health and contraceptive services.

The new program is reported to have already had an impact. Linking introduction of new methods to quality of care has precipitated service improvements in some sites, and participatory approaches have established broad-based, ongoing dialogue among stakeholders. In the latter respect, the objectives of the program are similar to those described for Reproductive Health Technologies' "Boom and Bust Initiative." While the presentation did not propose that this new strategy would be a panacea, it did conclude that the approach has so far proven fresh and valid. Presenter and participants agreed that the main challenges to expanding and replicating the program would be money, time, and sustainability.

A "Government Standards Defense"[*]

In its 1996 report,[30] the IOM committee reiterated the recommendation of the 1990 National Research Council/IOM contraceptive research and development committee that the U.S. Congress enact a federal product liability statute that would make FDA approval of contraceptive drugs and devices available to contraceptive manufacturers as a defense against punitive damages, assuming proper compliance with FDA regulatory requirements. Both committees contended that, for controversial products that contribute importantly to the public health yet produce only modest profit margins, limits on liability could act as an incentive for research and development or at least could reduce the amount of disincentive. The 1990 committee argued that pharmaceuticals and medical devices are unique among products in the United States in the degree to which quality is regulated before they are released in the market, so that the need for liability as a quality control mechanism is greatly reduced.

As conceptualized by that committee, with such a statute—variously referred to as a federal, government, or regulatory standards defense; regulatory approval or compliance defense; or simply as an "FDA defense"—companies would not be held liable for punitive damages in a lawsuit under the following assumptions: if the drug or medical device involved had received approval from the FDA and if that company had fully complied with all of the agency's requirements for premarketing testing and postmarketing surveillance. The defense would not, however, bar plaintiffs from obtaining full compensatory and noneconomic damages. Nor would it be available to a manufacturer found to have withheld from the FDA either information gathered for purposes of premarketing approval, or information developed after approval for review so as to determine whether the product in question, its marketing, or its labeling should be modified. In other words, a consumer injured by a hazard that otherwise would have been discovered would not be barred from suit should a company have failed to comply with FDA requirements.

The presenter's response to the query posed by the subcommittee as to whether some kind of federal standards defense might have "made a difference" in Norplant's legal and market experience was that it might well have constituted a substantial deterrent. The contingency is that the claims related to Norplant have been for relatively modest injuries, that is, modest compared to such serious injuries as birth defects, which would have been likely to generate suits in any event.

---

[*]See Appendix A, *Presentation 15* (Green).

The principal issues proposed in this presentation for advancing thought about the potential and feasibility of some sort of regulatory approval defense in connection with contraceptives are: FDA capacity for serving as the anchor for such a defense, the related matter of postmarketing surveillance, the question of whether such a defense would actually have the stimulating effect on industry research and development that has been widely hypothesized, the instruction that can be had in this connection from the experience of those U.S. states that have enacted product liability legislation, and the most politically feasible scope of a government standards defense.

FDA's capabilities for fulfilling its responsibilities during the premarketing period are substantial, but the postmarketing period is more problematic. The 1990 IOM committee spoke frankly on the inadequacy of existing postmarketing surveillance systems for contraceptive products and on the ethical, practical, and economic obstacles to successful postmarketing surveillance, and recommended establishment of a comprehensive system to provide systematic and timely feedback about both the positive and negative health effects of contraceptive products. Both IOM committees noted that because a regulatory standards defense would necessarily interact with postmarketing surveillance efforts, any recommendation for such a statute would be more compelling were formal postmarketing surveillance studies to be an integral and general requirement.

As for the general wisdom that liability relief would be an incentive to contraceptive research and development, the proof that it has been a disincentive cannot be gotten through any retrospective study that could be called scientific, so that it must be tested prospectively in the doing. There is, however, useful instruction to be had from the experience with state-level legislation and the relevant, though imperfectly applicable, attempts in the fields of aviation and vaccines to test hypotheses about the causal relationship between product liability and industrial research and development.

Finally, and related to all of the above, is the scope of a defense that would be politically imaginable, critical to which would be a purposive and meticulous analysis of legislative experience in this area to date.

3

Workshop Summary and Analysis

This workshop arose from the belief that reviewing the experience with the development and introduction of the contraceptive implant, Norplant, would be illuminating. As the first real contraceptive innovation in over two decades and as a long-acting method requiring clinical intervention for its application and removal, the method raised a range of issues that could offer valuable lessons about the challenges to be addressed if other new technologies are to enter the contraceptive marketplace, so as to make the entry of those technologies as positive and trouble-free as possible.

The workshop had three objectives:

- to review newly available data on Norplant's efficacy, safety, and use;
- to extract lessons from diverse aspects of the method's development, introduction, use, and market experience; and
- to explore approaches to developing and introducing new contraceptives based on learning from the Norplant market experience.

The workshop consisted of these elements: 17 formal presentations; two organized dialogues, one on consumer perspectives, the other on strategies for developing and introducing new contraceptive technologies; and extensive discussion among subcommittee members, presenters, and invited participants on the information presented and its implications. The dialogues were led by panels of individuals with perspectives from women's health advocacy, reproductive ethics, and the clinic. The subcommittee then met in executive session to analyze the workshop proceedings and develop a list of lessons and points for further consideration or action.

The following section presents:

- a data review, consisting of brief summary statements on key points presented at the workshop;
- the subcommittee's analysis of those lessons learned that it considered most crucial for the future; and
- areas for consideration and action.

DATA REVIEW

Efficacy

Data were presented from two 5-year-long studies of major short- to medium-term side effects of implant contraceptives not identified in clinical trials: the Postmarketing Surveillance of Norplant led by WHO and pre-introductory studies led by the Population Council. The evidence from those studies was that both Norplant and the two-rod levonorgestrel implant system are highly efficacious, with failure rates under 1 percent per year, thus providing reversible contraceptive protection essentially equal to that of permanent methods, that is, tubal ligation and vasectomy.

Safety

As with all hormonal methods, the contraceptive implant is unsuitable for some women and those contraindications are detailed in its labeling. The Postmarketing Surveillance and Population Council studies found serious adverse events to be extremely rare among implant users over 5 years of study and concluded that, in the settings where those studies were carried out, the method proved to be safe and well-tolerated.

The studies presented at the workshop on the biocompatibility of the polymer known as "silicone rubber" used in the implant produced the following information. First, while the capsules do provoke a typical local foreign-body reaction, the character of the biomaterial and its interface with tissue are not associated with pathological problems. Second, the silicone gel in breast implants is not the same, chemically or biologically, as the silicone rubber used in Norplant, and there are no data that indicate that the silicone elastomer used in Norplant acts as an adjuvant that could potentiate autoimmune disease.

A question that has been asked about the safety of the hormonal implant is whether its progesterone-like effect might, in human beings, produce the same thinning of vaginal epithelium and increased transmission of immunodeficiency virus effected in a monkey model. The report to the workshop was that at present, the quality of the available data does not permit any such conclusions but that until better human studies become available, clinical management of high-risk clients should emphasize protection from sexually transmitted infections through condom use and other safe sexual practices, with optimal contraceptive protection accorded secondary priority.

User Profiles

The characteristics of the women in international samples differed too substantially from country to country to permit easy generalizations. In the United States, the 1995 National Survey of Family Growth points to two groups of Norplant users. The largest consists of predominantly young, single, minority women of lower socioeconomic status and educational levels, with one or more children, less likely to live in rural areas or in the northeastern portion of the country, and using the method primarily for spacing. A smaller group of older women of higher parity appears to be adopting the method as a long-term reversible alternative to tubal ligation.

Side Effects

Contraceptive implants produce side effects for many women, as described in the product labeling. By far the most common are changes in menstrual patterns, predominantly prolonged or irregular menstrual flow or increased bleeding. These tend to be frequent during the first 6 to 9 months of use, stabilizing by the end of the first year at a level that becomes acceptable to a majority of continuing users. The method also has nonmenstrual side effects which manifest with different frequency and relative importance in different populations and at different time points, but primarily include headache, vaginal discharge, weight gain, acne, pelvic pain, and mood alterations. The studies presented suggest that the simple presence of menstrual side effects does not reliably predict decisions to continue or discontinue implant use, but there are differences between continuers and discontinuers with respect to nonmenstrual side effects. Discontinuation rates associated with nonmenstrual side effects seem higher than those for menstrual side effects but no single side effect, menstrual or nonmenstrual, is consistently associated with decisions to discontinue use.

Continuation and Discontinuation

In studies to compare method use, implant continuation rates tend to be high relative to those of other reversible contraceptives. The overall pattern is that continuation rates are generally high through the first 2 years of use and not strikingly dissimilar from sample to sample, except in those studies that found discontinuation correlated with negative media coverage. Although there are great differences by country and although the data for the United States are scanty (partly because of low utilization), by the end of Norplant's approved 5-year term of use, approximately one-half of those who originally chose it were continuing use, with a significant proportion of those who discontinued having done so to start a pregnancy. And while explicitly comparative data are also scant, continuation rates for the implant are high compared to those for other reversible methods.

Much remains to be understood before making broad assertions about reasons for continuing and discontinuing use of the contraceptive implant and about how those reasons differ from population to population over the reproductive cycle. Menstrual disturbances and other medical reasons are undeniably important yet, overall, reasons for retaining or removing Norplant are a complex blend of personal experience of side effects, "other-directed" variables like the wishes of partners, and broader social influences, the passage of time, and changes in life plans. At least some women who stay with Norplant seem motivated to trade off side effects, even when burdensome in number or severity, for the convenience and efficacy they believe essential to greater control over their lives.

User Satisfaction

Information on user satisfaction is scarce. Data from clinic-based studies presented at the workshop found most women continuing Norplant use to be very satisfied with the method, while noting that they had not found it easy to get used to; their satisfaction level was slightly below satisfaction levels for Depo-Provera and the pill. The large majority of women continuing Norplant use would recommend it to others, a slightly smaller majority than for the other two methods but still high. Perceptions among those discontinuing use were much less positive: Very few of those discontinuing use indicated that they had been "very satisfied," compared to sizable minorities of those who had discontinued use of Depo-Provera and the pill. Both women continuing use and those discontinuing saw the best features of Norplant as its convenience and effectiveness; fewer Depo-Provera and pill-users, whether they were continuing use or had discontinued, cited those attributes as those methods' best features.

Postmarketing Surveillance

The report from the 5-year Postmarketing Surveillance of Norplant confirmed its value not only as a source of knowledge on adverse effects that cannot be identified in clinical trials, but as evidence that large-scale, longer-term surveillance studies using cohort methodology can now be considered feasible in developing countries.

Cost-Effectiveness

A "savings" model indicated that all forms of contraception, including dual-method use, are far less costly in the United States than an unintended pregnancy. In that array, the implant was shown to rank very high in terms of cost-effectiveness compared to other contraceptive methods, saving almost $14,000 over a 5-year period of use.

In sum, no good scientific reasons emerged in the workshop for not making Norplant available to all women for whom its use is not counterindicated in labeling.

LESSONS LEARNED

In its post-workshop analysis of the workshop proceedings, the subcommittee was struck by the amount of agreement on the overarching lessons from the Norplant experience. Variability in workshop participants' perspectives on those issues were differences of emphasis, for example, what had mattered most or first in the sequence of events involving the method. Yet, at end of day, views on what is needed for the future were not widely disparate, although differences can be expected around implementation practicalities, roles and responsibilities, and financing. While some of the lessons may be particular to long-acting contraceptive methods, they are not exclusive to such methods and still point clearly to areas where there are lessons to be applied to the development and introduction of new contraceptive technologies as a general matter. In fact, a primary value of the workshop was that it effectively named the issues to be put promptly on the table as preparation for the next contraceptive, as both cautionary and positive guidance.

The full committee's extensive analysis of the field of contraceptive research and development, which culminated in its 1996 report, led to some conclusions that are appropriately repeated here as preface to this report's closing sections. First, while contraception is frequently used and new contraceptive technologies seem to be much needed and desired, as an area of human health it has certain intrinsic complexities. Perhaps the most important of these are that contraceptives are used, often for long periods of time, by presumably healthy individuals, who are less inclined to accept limitations and side effects. Second, contraception is also closely linked to social, cultural, and personal norms and values that, varying by setting, require considerable sensitivity. Third, the likelihood in the foreseeable future of a single contraceptive that will be perfect for all potential users across their lifetimes, totally effective yet totally free of side effects, is small. Fourth, like all pharmaceuticals, the development, production, and distribution of contraceptives are in varying ways connected to, if not dependent on, a commercial market with needs and expectations that do not inevitably coincide with those of public health. Finally, the subcommittee concluded that just as there was no single prime cause for the difficulties that have surfaced regularly in the field of contraceptive research and development and which have had such impact on Norplant's experience, there is no single, prime solution for those difficulties.

TABLE 3-1 Lessons Learned

The Delivery Side of the Health Care Equation Is a Commanding Factor

The principal lesson concerning Norplant was that when used in a medically controlled environment, it proved to be a highly effective and safe contraceptive method, responsive to the needs of significant numbers of women. However, as the most technologically complex contraceptive method so far introduced onto the market and as one dependent for its provision on health care systems, Norplant's utilization in large populations was never going to be simple, even though its introduction had been preceded by many years of basic and clinical research. Like all the most effective contraceptives now on the market, the method was designed to be applied in contexts requiring specific standards and, as the most technologically challenging of those methods, it demanded authentic competence in a minor surgical procedure in a clinic setting of good quality. These optimal contexts were not always secured: Extension of the method from limited populations to larger domestic and international settings was associated with shortcomings in application that confounded the value of the method with the quality of its delivery. The great preponderance of the method's difficulties were those that have to do with larger, systemic difficulties in assuring provider training and evidence of competency, delivery system capacity for assuring the quality of all required services, the adequacy and appropriateness of counseling and communication, and the character and timing of consumer involvement.

Providing and Receiving Training in New Contraceptive Methods Are Equally Critical

Complicated implant removals were the basis, in 1994, of the first lawsuit involving Norplant and the subsequent flood of media coverage and litigation. This occurred despite the efforts by the method's distributors and nonprofit intermediaries to train large numbers of providers in the technology. Those efforts were affected by a range of factors, each discussed in the course of the workshop and reflected in this report in the section on "Training for Insertion and Removal," including, most importantly:

- fast, high-volume program takeoff;
- insufficient appreciation of the importance of proper insertions for easier removals;
- limited practice in removal technique and predicting and preparing for complications;
- lack of participation in training on the part of some providers who did insertions;
- health care system structures that made uniformity of practice and assurance of competence difficult; and
- insufficient sensitivity to the social, cultural, and personal dimensions of contraception, especially those particular to long-acting, "provider-dependent" contraceptives.

The workshop material provided by presenters indicated that approximately 95 percent of removals were successful and without significant problems. While these were research sites and might be expected to have higher success rates, they indicate a potential that can be achieved and possibly improved.

Continued

TABLE 3-1 *Continued*

Counseling and Communication Are Pivotal

Case material indicated that intensive counseling was associated with better acceptance and continuation rates, partly because women deciding to use the contraceptive implant were carefully identified at the outset, partly because they were provided with enough information to choose freely, and partly because they acquired more complete understanding of what to expect in the form of side effects. There is anecdotal evidence that clinical response to management of side effects was less evenly successful and that women's concerns about side effects were sometimes not given proper attention. The lesson here is a description of what communication about contraceptive choice would ideally be: a continuum spanning appropriate and intelligible product labeling; adequate provider training, collaboration between provider and client at the point of method choice; and support for clients in dealing with side effects and possible discontinuation, all the way to removal on demand or as approved efficacy ends and a new contraceptive choice must be made. This would optimally occur as truly two-way dialogue; information exchanged and necessary understandings would be complete and unconstrained by time; dialogue would be ongoing across the full course of contraceptive use; client participation in contraceptive choice would be truly voluntary; and the hierarchical distinctions between provider and client would be muted to the extent necessary for all this to happen.

Taking Context into Careful Account Is Essential

Experience with Norplant highlighted the fact that long-acting, provider-dependent contraceptive methods require special regard to ensure that decisions for their election and continued use are freely made and well informed. Failures in this respect not only have ethical implications but more broadly affect the proper utilization of the technology in question and its reputation. For example, although all such efforts failed, legislative and judicial attempts made in the United States to use Norplant coercively were perceived by some panelists and the constituencies they represented as evocative of some past attempts to restrict reproductive freedom that had disproportionately affected minority women. This had added to a residue of suspicion and affected objective assessment of the method. Lack of free choice, in method election and continuation, was also an issue in some developing countries, where it also led to negative public perceptions of the method overall, thus discouraging its use for many women for whom it would have been appropriate.

Costs Matter

The topic of cost-effectiveness raised questions for further consideration, importantly the meaning of costs, to both consumers and providers, for contraceptive availability and utilization. Real or imagined costs did act as barriers to Norplant use, notably in connection with removal for some women in some clinics. Workshop participants agreed that the entire subject of costs requires more creative thinking—about the cost of the method and its financing, about how to assure removal, and about clear policies of removal upon demand that are more effectively communicated to women considering the method.

NEXT STEPS: AREAS FOR CONSIDERATION AND ACTION

In analyzing what learning from Norplant's experience indicated for the future, the subcommittee identified nine areas for further consideration or action that could conceivably make the terrain for new or improved contraceptive technologies more hospitable than has been the case for Norplant. Of those areas, some are matters of broad context, while others relate to specific parts of the processes of contraceptive research, development, and introduction. Some would expand or deepen work now informed by that experience; others would involve new effort. Together, these areas can be viewed as critical pieces of a strategy whose most immediate application might be to the introduction of other implant formulations and, later, to the full span of the development and introduction of any new contraceptive technology.

The text that follows presents these areas in two groups. The first consists of areas where the science indicates that more answers are needed or where strengthening or expansion would build on the positive learning from the Norplant experience. The second group consists of areas in which the Norplant experience revealed clear deficits and where new and, in some cases, bold initiatives will be critical for a different future. The subcommittee offers all these elements as options and propositions for further discussion, consensus-building, and action—signposts on the way forward.

Areas for Strengthening or Expansion

1. Clinical Research

Data reported at the workshop pointed to two areas where more fundamental research is needed to strengthen the position of implantable contraceptives in the array of contraceptive options:

• research on vaginal response to hormones, including cyclic hormonal effects, and on the use of progestins in contraceptives on the incidence of sexually transmitted disease, importantly including HIV; and
• research on the causes of hormonal side effects that, in addition to their implications for the users of hormonal methods, also affect the ability of providers to manage and treat those events clinically.

2. Market Research

In its 1996 report, the full IOM committee* concluded that the clear priorities in the "women's agenda" set forth at the 1994 International Conference on Population and Development, along with dramatic advances in the science that make response to those priorities far more feasible, add new dimensions to the landscape for contraceptive and anti-infective research and development. However, implementing an agenda driven more intensely by what women want underscores the importance of fortifying pioneering efforts to engage consumers much earlier than has been customary, doing more with the kinds of research typical of commercial markets, and proceeding in as cross-sectoral a manner as possible. To do that would require development of more explicit and systematic public-sector strategies for:

- early, purposive, and systematic interactions among product developers and marketers, nonprofit intermediaries, and representatives from key consumer and provider groups, beginning with product design and subsequently at key points in the development, preintroductory, and introductory phases; and
- utilization of a full range of quantitative and qualitative market research techniques throughout.

3. "Preintroduction"

Three consecutive sets of experience with Norplant's introduction, each building somewhat on the one before, highlighted the many utilities of inserting what amounts to a "preintroductory" phase that permits various assessments prior to full-scale product introduction, thus diminishing possibilities of later difficulties.

"Introduction" was thoughtfully utilized by the Population Council as a bridge from research and development and from the successful completion of clinical trials, to Norplant's entry into national family planning programs. The key mechanism was introductory trials in a limited set of facilities that then became centers for extension of training after national product registration; their purpose was to identify management and technical issues affecting method delivery and to develop and refine guidelines, standards, counseling materials, and training programs for clinical management. In the United Kingdom, the principal mechanism was premarket research focused on provider attitudes and delivery system issues that might present problems, in order to take those into account in training and actual scaled-up introduction. The WHO Strategic Approach then significantly expanded such preintroductory questions by stepping back and asking first whether a new method should be introduced at all in certain countries until the

---

*The references made in this section to "the Committee" are to the Institute of Medicine's Committee on Contraceptive Research and Development and its full report on the state of the field (see Endnote 1).

necessary systems are strengthened sufficiently to accommodate the addition of a new technology.

The WHO Approach has three stages, the first proceeding to the next only when and if the decision is made to introduce the new method:

• Stage 1: assessment of need, in a specific country family planning program, for an additional contraceptive technology, including initial assessment of existing method mix, service infrastructure and capability, program policies, potential user demand, cost-benefit to user/program, and logistics management.
• Stage 2: introductory trial, service delivery research, and user perspective research, in an integrated sequence.
• Stage 3: analysis and participatory review of research results, decision-making on next steps, and strategy development.

The subcommittee, while mindful of the issues of cost, time, and sustainability attached to adopting this strategy as a standard approach, regards this three-stage framework as "best practice" for the future, with further experience expected to make such processes more efficient.

4. Informed Decision-Making

Informed decision-making is a general concern for the clinical management of any new medical technology, but the Norplant experience underscored the fact that all long-acting, provider-dependent contraceptives have special characteristics and therefore require special attention. The questions the workshop participants flagged as of greatest concern were:

• how mechanisms for informed decision-making are to be developed and by whom;
• the distinctions and connections among the kinds of information needed in the experimental stages of product development, compared to what is needed in the introductory phases and in routine clinic settings;
• the purposes and practical implications of labeling, informed consent documents, and clinical guidelines for informational and decision-making purposes;
• what is essential as opposed to discretionary information; and
• the impact of all the above on participation in contraceptive research and development.

If and when new long-acting, provider-dependent contraceptive products are developed and introduced, each of these concerns would ideally be part of a systematic strategy for informed decision-making, to then be tested and refined in the product's clinical trial and preintroductory phases. The subcommittee felt that development of core guidelines and clinical materials for possible new products would be an effective way to catalyze and focus the necessary thinking about these concerns, as well as any potential areas of difficulty, in an organized and concrete way.

5. Postmarketing Surveillance

The concerted public-sector effort to carry out postmarketing surveillance underscored the value of such surveillance as a source of knowledge of adverse effects that cannot be identified in clinical trials. It also proved that such studies are feasible in developing countries. Postmarketing surveillance might also become an integral component of new product liability legislation. At the same time, such surveillance adds to costs which, in the case of Norplant, were defrayed by the World Health Organization and private foundations. This raises a general question about future financial support for such studies by the public sector, as well as a specific question about the responsibility for financing them were they to be required as a component of a federal standards defense. Both need to be addressed.

Areas for New Initiative

6. Credentialing

A significantly problematic aspect to Norplant's introduction derived from the fact that requirements for reasonable competence in surgical procedure are uneven across clinical facilities worldwide. This is especially problematic when new technologies are introduced rapidly, as was the case with Norplant despite major investment in provider training. While this situation is likely to persist, it could be susceptible to a thoughtful, individual-case approach. Accordingly, the subcommittee concluded from the workshop discussions that collaboration with professional medical societies and major managed care organizations on strategies for training and assuring provider competence would be a critical preparatory step in introducing the next new provider-dependent contraceptive technology, most immediately the LNG two-rod implant.

7. Core Guidelines for Long-Acting Contraceptives

A key to any serious attempt to implement informed decision-making in clinical situations is helping providers to actually make it possible. This suggested to the subcommittee that a most effective route to such implementation would be, again, to enlist the cooperation of the pertinent professional medical societies. The tasks would be to develop a collaboration among representation from those societies and a range of consumer groups to recruit necessary additional expertise, and to work on fashioning core guidelines for the introduction and clinical management of long-acting contraceptives. Addressing the potential for inappropriate use and how to prevent it would be an integral component. An ancillary task would be development of a strategy for dissemination of those guidelines in the corresponding professional communities. These core guidelines could then be modified culturally or linguistically for specific populations as needed.

While such guidelines would be particularly important for introducing long-acting contraceptives into contexts where past attempts to use such methods had been problematic, they would also be valuable for introducing any new contraceptive method into environments where educational level, language, culture, or socioeconomic status have the potential to constrain well-informed decision-making.

8. Costs

Real or imagined costs did act as barriers to Norplant use, notably in connection with removal for some women in some clinics. Systematic understanding of the effects of price on initial adoption is lacking. At the same time, in the subcommittee's view, Norplant's history raises a separate and complicated question that is likely to arise in the future. That question is how to develop pricing structures in cases where a large proportion of R&D costs have been borne by the public and quasi-public sectors, at the same time that industry profit requirements and risk exposure are appropriately taken into account.

The issues around Norplant's costs raise other issues that merit prompt and systematic analysis and discussion that is focused on actionable outcomes:

- public-sector cost constraints;
- political and economic tensions around tiered pricing structures;
- the role of health insurance coverage of contraception and health plan formularies;
- diversification and expansion of the market for contraceptives in general; and
- different meanings of cost-effectiveness for consumers, countries at varying levels of development, and delivery systems.

Each has implications for what constitutes a market share that might be appealing to industrial investment as contraceptives grow in variety and, as Norplant user profiles suggest, may increasingly become niche products.

9. Product Liability

The Norplant experience provides further grounds for the perception that product liability, or simply the anticipation of liability, stifles industrial investment in development of new contraceptives. The most immediate example is the fact that the improved two-rod, three-year implant that is significantly easier to insert and remove is not being introduced in the United States by its European manufacturers, apparently owing to litigation concerns related to Norplant, so that it may not become available as a contraceptive option for American women. A related concern is the current controversy around silicone products and its potential effects on the supply of biomaterial not only for implant contraceptives but for other medical devices, some of which—for example, cerebrospinal fluid shunt systems and pacemaker leads—are essential to life.

The subcommittee and workshop participants again voiced support for the conclusion of the 1990 and 1996 Institute of Medicine committees concerning the potential importance of enactment of a product liability statute. Broadly stated, such a statute would make FDA approval of contraceptive drugs and devices available to manufacturers as a defense against punitive damages, assuming proper compliance with FDA regulatory requirements. The subcommittee recognizes that the complexities and ramifications of a defense of this nature are many, so that a crucial—and urgent—area of work will be systematic, very practical conceptualization of alternative configurations of such a defense as a foundation for possible legislative work.

FINAL COMMENT

The purpose of this workshop was to learn from the many years of intersectoral activity dedicated to the development and introduction of Norplant. The fact of emphasis on barriers and problems should not obscure the considerable positive learning from the Norplant experience that, consolidated and refined, can only make the advent of new contraceptives smoother.

At the same time, there were social and cultural aspects of Norplant's market experience that were negative to an extent that overwhelmed the best of those efforts. Some of these aspects will change slowly, if at all; others may be at least partly susceptible to new areas of initiative discussed in the workshop and highlighted in the preceding section. A pivotal challenge will be determining how those initiatives are to be pursued and by whom.

The workshop participants and the subcommittee agreed that contraceptive research and development have fallen behind in the great advances propelling the rest of medicine, including all other areas of women's health, and that, without attention to these areas of major impediment, contraceptives will continue to compete poorly when industries contemplate alternative new directions for their investment portfolios. They agreed as well with the conclusion of the full Committee "that there is not likely to be a 'silver bullet' solution to the dilemmas faced by the field of contraceptive research and development. Each piece of the dilemma will have to be tackled in cumulative fashion as part of a coherent strategy, each resolution improving matters somewhat and eventually amassing enough weight to tip the balance in a more positive direction."

ENDNOTES

1. Institute of Medicine. Contraceptive Research and Development: Looking to the Future. PF Harrison, A Rosenfield, eds. Washington, D.C.: National Academy Press, 1996. The study was supported by the Rockefeller Foundation, the Andrew W. Mellon Foundation, the National Institute of Child Health and Human Development, the Contraceptive Research and Development (CONRAD) Program, and the United States Agency for International Development.

2. The workshop and this report are supported by a grant from the Henry J. Kaiser Family Foundation.

3. Medical officer NDA review. NDA#19-897. Rockville, MD: Food and Drug Administration, 1990. — Grubb GS, D Moore, NG Anderson, et al. Pre-introductory clinical trials of Norplant® implants: A comparison of 17 countries' experience. *Contraception* 52:287–296, 1995. — Sivin I. Contraception with NORPLANT® implants. *Human Reproduction* 9:1818–1826, 1994.

4. Patient labeling for Norplant is organized by risks, warning signals, precautions, and side effects. Provider prescribing information is organized by contraindications, warnings, precautions, and adverse reactions. For Norplant, the FDA sorted the last group into four subcategories: (a) conditions associated with Norplant during the first year of use; (b) conditions that occurred more frequently among Norplant users than among a control group of IUD users, with differences in incidence great enough to attain statistical significance as being probably related to Norplant use; (c) conditions occurring with a frequency of 5 percent or more during the first year of use in clinical trials and judged to have possibly been associated with its use; and (d) conditions observed in Norplant users postmarketing but for which there is no basis for judging a causal relationship (Food and Drug Administration. Norplant® Implants Revised Labeling: Information for Providers [Draft], March 1995).

5. Affandi B, SSI Santoso, Djajadilaga, W Hadisaputra, FA Moeloek, J Prihartono, F Lubis, and RS Samil. Five-year experience with NORPLANT. *Contraception* 36:417–428, 1987.

Akhter H, TR Dunson, RN Amatya, K Begum, T Chowdhury, N Dighe, SL Krueger, and S Rahman. A five-year clinical evaluation of NORPLANT contraceptive subdermal implants in Bangladesh acceptors. *Contraception* 47:569–582, 1993.

Brache V, F Alvarez-Sanchez, A Faundes, AS Tejeda, and L Cochon. Free levonorgestrel index and its relationship to luteal activity during long-term use of NORPLANT implants. *Advances in Contraception* 8:319–326, 1992.

Chompootaweep S, E Kochagarn, S Sirisumpan, J Tang-ushu, B Teppitaksak, and N Dusitin. Effectiveness of NORPLANT implants among Thai women in Bangkok. *Contraception* 53:33–36, 1996.

Crosby UD, BE Schwarz, KL Gluck, and SF Heartwell. A preliminary report of NORPLANT implant insertions in a large urban family planning program. *Contraception* 48:359–366, 1993.

Cullins VE, PD Blumenthal, RE Remsburg, and GR Huggins. Preliminary experience with NORPLANT in an inner-city population. *Contraception* 47:193–204, 1993.

Cullins VE, RE Remsburg, PD Blumenthal, et al. Comparison of adolescent and adult experiences with Norplant levonorgestrel contraceptive implants. *Obstetrics and Gynecology* 83:1026–1032, 1994.

Diaz S, HB Croxatto, M Pavez, H Belhadj, J Stern, and I Sivin. Clinical assessment of treatment for prolonged bleeding in users of NORPLANT implants. *Contraception* 42:97–110, 1990.

Diaz S, M Pavez, P Miranda, DN Robertson, I Sivin, and HB Croxatto. A five-year clinical trial of levonorgestrel silastic implants (NORPLANT). *Contraception* 25:447–456, 1982.

Frank ML, AN Poindexter III, LM Cornin, CA Cox, and L Bateman. One-year experience with subdermal contraceptive implants in the United States. *Contraception* 48:229–249, 1993.

Gabrielle CA, WM O'Fallon, LT Kurland, CM Beard, JE Woods, and J Melton III. Risk of connective-tissue diseases and other disorders after breast implantation. *New England Journal of Medicine* 330:1697–1702, 1994.

Grubb G, D Moore, NG Anderson, et al. Pre-introductory clinical trials of NORPLANT implants: A comparison of 17 countries' experience. *Contraception* 52:287–296, 1995.

Gu S-J, I Sivin, M-K Du, L-D Zhang, L-R Ying, F Meng, S-L Wu, P-Z Wang, Y-L Gao, X He, L-F Qi, C-R Chen, Y-P Liu, and D Wang. Effectiveness of NORPLANT implants through seven years, a large-scale study in China. *Contraception* 52:99–103, 1995.

Gu S-J, M-K Du, L-D Zhang, Y-L Liu, S-H Wang, and I Sivin. A 5-year evaluation of NORPLANT contraceptive implants in China. *Obstetrics and Gynecology* 83:673–678, 1994.

Indian Council for Medical Research (ICMR) Task Force on hormonal contraception. *Contraception* 48:1230–1232, 1993.

Koetsawang S. The injectable contraceptive: Present and future trends. *In Frontiers in Human Reproduction*, M Seppala and L Hamberger, eds. pp. 30–42, The New York Academy of Sciences, New York (Annals vol. 662), 1991.

Moreno L, and N Goldman. Contraceptive failure rates in developing countries: Evidence from the demographic and health surveys. *International Family Planning Perspectives* 17:44–49, 1991.

Noerpramana, NP. A cohort study of NORPLANT implant: Side effects and acceptance. *Advances in Contraception* 11:97–114, 1995.

Olsson SE, V Odlind, EDB Johansson, and M Nordstrom. Plasma levels of levonorgestrel and free levonorgestrel index in women using NORPLANT implants or two covered rods (NORPLANT 2). *Contraception* 35:215–228, 1987.

Peers T, JE Stevens, J Graham, and A Davey. Norplant implants in the UK: First-year continuation and removal. *Contraception* 53:345–352, 1996.

Salah M, A-G M Ahmed, M Abu-Eloyoun, and MM Shaaban. 5-year experience with NORPLANT implants in Egypt. *Contraception* 35:543–550, 1987.

Sanchez-Guerrero J, GA Colditz, EW Karlson, DJ Hunter, F Speizer, and MH Liang. Silicone breast implants and the risk of connective tissue diseases and symptoms. *New England Journal of Medicine* 332:1666–1670, 1995.

Singh K, OAC Viegas, YF Fong, and SS Ratnam. Acceptability of NORPLANT implants for fertility regulation in Singapore. *Contraception* 45:39–47, 1992.

Singh K, OAC Viegas, and SS Ratnam. Acceptability of NORPLANT 2 as a method of family planning. *Contraception* 45:453–461, 1992.

Sivin I. Contraception with NORPLANT implants. *Human Reproduction* 9:1818–1826, 1994.

Sivin I. International experience with NORPLANT and NORPLANT 2 contraceptives. *Studies in Family Planning* 19:81–94, 1988.

Tietze C, and S Lewit. Evaluation of intrauterine devices: Ninth progress report of the cooperative statistical program. *Studies in Family Planning* 1(55):1–40, 1970.

Trussell J, and K Kost. Contraceptive failure in the United States: A critical review of the literature. *Studies in Family Planning* 18:237–283, 1987.

Trussell J, JA Leveque, JD Koenig, R London, S Borden, J Hennebarry, KD LaGuardia, FH Stewart, TG Wilson, S Wysocki, and MJ Strauss. The economic value of contraception: A comparison of 15 methods. *American Journal of Public Health* 85:494–503, 1995.

Mosher WD, and CA Bachrach. Understanding United States fertility: Continuity and change in the National Survey of Family Growth, 1988–1995. *Family Planning Perspectives* 28:4–12, 1996.

World Health Organization. Multinational comparative clinical evaluation of two long-acting injectable steroids: Norethisterone oenanthate and medroxyprogesterone acetate use-effectiveness. *Contraception* 15:513–533, 1977.

6. The expected rate of ectopic pregnancy is derived from the rate for women who are using no formal contraceptive method but may be in lactational amenorrhea or at risk of pregnancy or pregnant following non-use. In the Postmarketing Surveillance, the rate has drifted down over the years from approximately 4 per 1,000 woman-years to a final value near 2 per 1,000, or 0.2 to 0.4 per 100 woman-years. In the U.S. population as a whole in the 1970s, the risk was 2.6 per 1,000 among non-users of contraceptives, according to estimates by the Centers for Disease Control and Prevention. Whatever value is used between 0.2 and 0.4 per 100, the relative risk to women in the Postmarketing Surveillance was only 1/7th to 1/13th of the risk of non-use of a contraceptive method. The far higher value of 0.13 per 100 in the U.S. label (written as 1.3 per 1,000 years) stems from the threefold higher pregnancy rate in the Population Council studies, a rate consequent to use of hard tubing in heavier-weight women.

7. Rose NR. The silicone breast implant controversy: The other courtroom. *Arthritis and Rheumatism* 39:615–618, 1996.

8. Naim JO, RJ Lanzafame, and CJ van Oss. The effect of silicone gel on the immune response. *Journal of Biomaterial Science: Polymer Edition* 7(2):123–132, 1995.

9. Freundlich N. Commentary: Congress should protect this medical lifeline. *Business Week*, 21 April 1997:120.

10. Marx PA, AI Spira, A Gettie, et al. Progesterone implants enhance SIV vaginal transmission and early virus load. *Nature/Medicine* 2:1084–1089, 1996.

11. The 1995 cycle of the NSFG gathered data between January and October 1995 on a national probability sample of women aged 15–44 selected from households followed by the National Health Interview Survey, a continuous multistage household survey. Numbers, percents, averages, and other statistics reported from the NSFG are weighted national estimates that account for different sampling rates and for nonresponse, and are adjusted to agree with control totals provided by the U.S. Bureau of the Census. The 10,847 women in the NSFG represent the 60.2 million women in the civilian noninstitutional population of the United States in 1995. Thus, on average, each woman in the NSFG represents about 5,500 women in that population.

12. According to NSFG data that became available after the workshop, 64.2 percent of the 60.2 million women aged 15–44 represented by the NSFG sample (N = 10,847) in 1995 were using contraception. Among those contraceptors, percentage distributions of use were as follows:

Female sterilization	17.8
Pill	17.3
Condom	13.1
Male sterilization	7.0
Withdrawal	2.0
Injectable	1.9
Periodic abstinence[a]	1.5
Diaphragm	1.2
Implant	0.9
Intrauterine device	0.5
Female condom	0.0
Other methods[b]	1.0

[a]Includes natural family planning (0.2 percent).
[b]Morning-after pill, foam, cervical cap, Today® sponge, suppository, jelly or cream (without diaphragm), and other methods not shown separately.

Abma J, A Chandra, W Mosher, L Peterson, and L Piccinino. Fertility, Family Planning, and Women's Health: New Data from the 1995 National Survey of Family Growth (*Vital and Health Statistics* 23[19]). Washington, D.C.: Centers for Disease Control and Prevention/National Center for Health Statistics, May 1997.

13. The Ortho Birth Control Studies are annual surveys by the Ortho Pharmaceutical Corporation of contraceptive attitudes and use. Random sampling is not employed and the surveys tend to underrepresent black women and households with annual incomes greater than $50,000.

14. The term "menstrual changes" is meant to express alterations in previous patterns and includes as most significant heavier menstrual flow, greater cycle irregularity, increased spotting, longer periods, and more painful periods.

15. According to NSFG data not available until after the workshop, as of 1995 4.5 percent of U.S. women aged 15–44 had ever used Depo-Provera and 1.9 percent were current users; those figures for Norplant use were 2.1 percent and 0.9 percent, respectively (Abma et al., *op. cit.*, 1997).

16. Preliminary figures were presented at the workshop in support of the assertions in this paragraph but, at the time this report went to press, final figures could not be released for formal publication.

17. The text of the recommendation reads as follows: "The committee recommends that, to make a full range of contraceptive products accessible to consumers and to increase demand for contraceptive products to something closer to the level of unmet need, there should be continued and sufficient government support of contraceptives services—for males as well as females—particularly for low-income individuals and particularly in developing countries. The committee also recommends that third-party payers, who bear the

costs and may reap the benefits of the health status of their covered populations, include contraception as a covered service. Ideally, family planning services and the management of sexual health would be integrated components of comprehensive reproductive health services" (Institute of Medicine, *op. cit.*, 1996).

18. The average wholesale price of Norplant in the United States is $365 for a kit containing the six capsules, trocar, scalpel, forceps, syringes and syringe needles, skin closure, gauze sponges, stretch bandage, and surgical drapes. Implantation and removal costs bring the total to about $700. At the 1995 World Bank consultation on the status of Norplant (World Bank/Population Council/World Health Organization Special Program on Research, Development, and Research Training in Human Reproduction. International Consultation on Contraceptive Implants, 19 July 1996 [unpublished paper]. Washington, DC: World Bank, 1995), the observation was made by one of the authors of the original contraceptive cost-effectiveness analysis (Trussell) that the savings model should be considered situational. For example, it cannot be calculated in the same way for developing countries, where the costs of unintended pregnancy—the chief driver for the model—may be valued differently, and where epidemiological factors differ. The price of the basic commodity also varies; the average Norplant kit price to developing country programs is $23. To that must be added public-sector health system costs for public education, training, supervision, implantation, and removal, a sizable commitment in the aggregate for donors providing commodity and/or program support and for countries with constrained health sector budgets.

19. From the beginning, patient labeling counseled women that while the implant should be removed at the end of 5 years when it would become less effective, it could be removed at any time before then, should the user wish to stop use for any reason (Wyeth-Ayerst Research Laboratories. Norplant® System Patient Labeling. Issued 10 December 1990.)

20. Just as this report was going to press, the following results, highly germane to this report, became available from a Population Council study of a representative sample of 2,979 current and former Norplant users in 14 Indonesian provinces:

(1.) No sizable removal backlog exists as was feared, owing to the fact that nurse/midwives had performed a large number of removals, although it was illegal for them to do so at the time, so that undercounting of completed removals and overcounting of pending removals were substantial.

(2.) Of the 8 percent of the sample who had not yet had their implants removed, 26 percent saw removal cost as an obstacle. About 91 percent of the women who had had implants removed underwent the procedure immediately on request; 9 percent encountered delay and resistance.

(3.) Most Norplant users obtained removals between the end of the fifth and end of the sixth year of use. Over 66 percent had continued to use the method for a full 5 years; 27 percent had undergone removal but then had a second Norplant set inserted. (Population Council News Release, 20 December 1997).

21. "Complication" as defined in the integrated summary of safety (NDA 19-897, Amendment 2) includes: multiple incisions; failure to remove implants completely, thereby requiring more than one additional visit; pain during removal; fainting; prolonged probing; or excessive time needed for removal.

22. Blumenthal PD, L Gaffikin, B Affandi, et al. Training for Norplant implant removal: Assessment of learning curves and competency. *Obstetrics and Gynecology* 89(2):174–178, February 1997.

23. Blumenthal PD, RE Remsburg, G Glew, et al. Usefulness of a clinical scoring system to anticipate difficulty of Norplant removal. *Advances in Contraception* 11:345–352, 1995.

24. The range in removal times has been found to be substantial. The multicentered Population Council trials found a fourfold variation by clinic from 4 to 17 minutes, with a coefficient of variation of about 50 percent in each clinic (Sivin I, O Viegas, I Campodonico, et al. Clinical performance of a new two-rod levonorgestrel contraceptive implant: A three-year randomized study with Norplant^R implants as controls. *Contraception* 55:73–80, February 1997).

25. Nearly two dozen bills in 13 states proposed variants on Norplant use in welfare cases and four women convicted of child abuse were ordered by courts to have Norplant inserted as a condition of probation (Davidson AR, and D Kalmuss. Topics for our times: Norplant coercion—An overstated threat. *American Journal of Public Health* 87[4]:550–551, April 1997). Two days after Norplant was approved by the FDA for distribution in the United States, an editorial in the *Philadelphia Inquirer* (Can contraception reduce the underclass? *Philadelphia Inquirer*, 12 December 1990: A18) elicited media commentary and public debate nationwide (SE Samuels, MD Smith, eds. *Dimensions of New Contraceptives: Norplant and Poor Women*. Menlo Park, CA: Henry J. Kaiser Family Foundation, 1992—Moskowitz EH, B Jennings, and D Callahan. Long-acting contraceptives: Ethical guidance for policymakers and health care providers. *Hastings Center Report 25*:1[Special Suppl], 1995.)

26. Walker KM. Judicial control of reproductive freedom: The use of Norplant as a condition of probation. 78 *Iowa Law Review* 779–812, 1993.

27. Roberts DE. Punishing drug addicts who have babies: Women of color, equality, and the right of privacy. 104 *Harvard Law Review* 1419, 1432 n.60, 1991.

28. Important among these is the Institute of Women and Ethnic Studies, a nonprofit, medical/community-based organization whose primary focus is the development of culturally proficient health intervention and research models. Its Women of Color Reproductive Health Forum held two workshops in 1996 that were pertinent to the work of the "Boom and Bust Initiative": *Finding Common Ground—Empowerment vs. Coercion—Long-Acting Contraceptives* (4–7 April 1996) and *Women of Color and the Emerging Health Technologies* (24–27 October 1996). The Institute has publicly stated its commitment to work with the Initiative, as well as with the Pacific Institute for Women's Health, to build consensus on culturally appropriate ethical approaches to reproductive health research, development, and marketing in order to expand the array of contraceptive options.

29. Bolivia, Brazil, Burkina Faso, Chile, Myanmar, South Africa, Vietnam, and Zambia.

30. Institute of Medicine, *op. cit.*, 1996.

Appendixes

A

Presentation Summaries

Presentation 1
WHAT INTERNATIONAL DATA TELL US NOW
Olav Meirik, M.D.
*World Health Organization,
Special Program of Research, Development, and
Research Training in Human Reproduction*

Background

This presentation reported provisional final results from the International Collaborative Postmarketing Surveillance led by the World Health Organization Special Program for Research, Development, and Research Training in Human Reproduction, with Family Health International and the Population Council. The purpose of the surveillance was to study, over a 5-year period, major short- to medium-term side effects of Norplant that had not been identified in clinical trials.

Methodology

The surveillance was based on a controlled concurrent cohort research design with a study population of women aged 18 to 40 at enrollment, and enrolled through a total of 32 family planning clinics in eight countries—Bangladesh, Chile, China, Colombia, Egypt, Indonesia, Sri Lanka, and Thailand. Index subjects were women choosing Norplant in those clinics, and controls age-matched by 5-year bands, who either chose intrauterine devices (IUDs) or sterilization. None had contraindications to Norplant or IUD use. The study population consisted of 7,977 Norplant acceptors (49.8%), 6,625 IUD acceptors (41.1%), and 1,419 sterilized women (8.9%), for a total of 16,021. The largest representation was from China: 6,114 participants, half of whom were Norplant acceptors.

The initial study objective was to have no more than 15 percent loss from enrollment, that is, a follow-up level of 85 percent. In fact, overall loss to follow-up over the course of the study was a much lower 3.6 percent: 0.1 percent in China, 7.6 percent in other Asian countries, 3.2 percent in Latin America, and 3.6 percent in Egypt. The study accumulated an average of approximately 4.8 calendar years of follow-up of IUD users, and 5 years of follow-up of both Norplant users and women who had been sterilized. The result was 78,000 woman-years of follow-up overall, 33,600 for current use of Norplant, 29,500 for IUDs, and 7,800 for sterilization.

Active follow-up continued for 5 years regardless of method changes and was carried out primarily through scheduled semi-annual visits, including home visits, letters, and telephone calls. Women were encouraged to come to the clinic if they had any health problems, and data from these unscheduled visits were recorded as well. In the case of inpatient care or outpatient clinic visits, records were retrieved and their content recorded. All major health-related events, significant health problems, and contact with health care services were recorded in personal diaries. "Major health-related events" included all deaths and hospitalizations, pregnancies, and morbidity and trauma that were potentially life-threatening, that required hospitalization and/or at least 1 month convalescence, that had long-term sequelae, or that required long-term medications.* "Significant health problems" were defined as virtually anything except common colds and minor injuries, all of which were reviewed by a country coordinator for purposes of standardization. Data were managed and coordinated centrally at WHO/HRP in Geneva, where they were reviewed, entered, and checked. All diagnoses were coded according to ICD-9 categories. Oversight included regular monitoring of clinics, site visits, and extensive correspondence with each clinic and collaborators in the study countries.

There were some methodological differences among clinics in assessment of side effects, so that some endpoints may reflect detection bias. For example, frequency of blood pressure checks varied by method use. Blood pressures for Norplant and IUD users were checked at least three times in about 40 percent and 31 percent of those two subpopulations respectively, in contrast to only 15 percent of the sterilized women. It may have been, however, that complaints of headaches among Norplant users led to more frequent blood pressure checks. Other possible sources of bias might be the frequency of hemoglobin measurements and overall numbers of visits. All such sources of bias are being analyzed further.

Findings

Age and Educational Levels

Overall, the majority of women in the study fell into the groups aged 24 to 35; however, women in China and Egypt tended to be older, with age distributions among the South American and Asian countries other than China roughly similar. As for education, those at the highest education levels chose the IUD, followed by Norplant, and then sterilization. The exception was South America, where the educational levels of Norplant and IUD users were almost identical.

---

*Results related to major health-related events were still provisional at the time of the workshop, because some analysis of individual diseases and conditions was still underway. After final review, there may be some reclassification of events.

Major Health-Related Events

There were 35 deaths in the course of this study, a rate of 0.44 per thousand woman-years. Just one of those was related to a reproductive event: a Sri Lankan woman who discontinued Norplant and became pregnant a year later, had a clandestine abortion, and died in sepsis.

Incidence of cardiovascular disease was in all cases below the power of the study. There were no cases of acute myocardial infarction. Three cases of stroke were recorded, two in China (one ischemic, one hemorrhagic) and one (unclassified) in Bangladesh 2 months after Norplant removal—a total of 3 per 100,000. There was one case of venous thromboembolism in a current Norplant user in Sri Lanka. Hypertension seemed somewhat more frequent in Norplant users than in the controls but, as indicated above, the extent to which this was a function of detection bias is unclear.

As for neoplastic disease, there were three confirmed cases of invasive breast cancer in current Norplant users and one in a current IUD user, all in China where the age distribution of the cohort in question would predict 2.8 cases over the same time period. There was one case of a clinically diagnosed metastatic breast cancer in a woman in Bangladesh who had used Norplant and oral contraceptives, and two cases of borderline breast malignancy (one phyllodes tumor and one *in situ* cancer), again, both in China. There was one case of invasive cervical cancer, diagnosed in Chile in a woman in the sterilization group. There were no cases of ovarian cancer.

Data were also gathered on diseases that have been associated with oral contraceptive use in general and that have also been addressed in studies of Norplant in the United States. These include gallbladder disease, found in 101 women, a rate of 1.28 per thousand woman-years, just slightly more frequent in Norplant users than in IUD users. As expected, in the 125 cases classified as anemias, incidence was highest among IUD users, lowest among women who had been sterilized. Diabetes mellitus, found in 12 subjects, was more frequent (eight cases) in Norplant users than in IUD users (three cases) or sterilization acceptors (one case), but the difference was not statistically significant.

Questions have been raised about a possible relationship between Norplant and systemic lupus erythematosus and collagen diseases, including rheumatoid arthritis and polyarthropathies. The frequencies encountered in the surveillance study samples were far too low to permit any conclusions: that is, three cases of lupus in China (two IUD users) and Egypt (one Norplant user), and nine cases of varying diagnoses of arthritis-related diseases, none long-term.

Significant Health-Related Problems

Included in this category were mood disturbances, anxiety, and depression; migraine or other headaches; and visual disturbances. Mood disturbances were recorded more frequently among Norplant users than among IUD users, but their incidence was similar to that generally found with other hormonal methods of contraception, mainly oral contraceptives. Incidences of these problems in IUD users and sterilized women were almost identical. Incidences of migraine and other headaches followed the same pattern.

As for visual disturbances, while there seemed to be higher incidence in Norplant users (19 cases, of which 15 were in Norplant users), closer scrutiny revealed no causal relationships. Six cases proved to be disorders of refraction, requiring eyeglasses; five cases were various diagnoses including borderline glaucoma, an intraocular foreign body, thyroiditis, cestode infection, and keratitis; and 8 cases (7 in Norplant users) were 1- to 3-month complaints associated with headache or fatigue, all reversible.

Continuation and Removals

The surveillance study was conducted in family planning clinics chosen for their good quality; all had had experience with Norplant and were familiar with both insertion and removal procedures, which may explain why continuation rates were so high and removal problems so few. Continuation rates for both Norplant and the IUD were exceptionally high: The cumulative 5-year continuation rate for Norplant was approximately 67 percent, for the IUD, 65 percent.

Out of 7,977 Norplant insertions, four were problematic (two each in two clinics). And, of the 7,827 removals that had occurred by 5 years of use, 79 had been difficult (10 per 1,000, or 1%), and 46 of those were in the same two clinics. "Difficult" was defined as cases involving broken capsules, removal requiring two sessions, or capsules that had been inserted too deeply. Since one of the clinics had been a training clinic, the question arises whether these difficult removals involved trainees. Both clinics are being evaluated.

Efficacy

Norplant has a very low contraceptive failure rate of 0.23 per 100 woman-years, compared to 0.15 for female sterilization. Norplant users were also found to be at very low risk of ectopic pregnancy, 0.03 per 100 woman-years, compared to a rate of 0.19 per 100 woman-years for non-contracepting women.

Conclusions

• Prospective postmarketing surveillance studies can now be said to be feasible in developing countries. Their considerable value does not exclude, however, the need for continued follow-up, particularly in the form of operational research.

- Norplant appears to have patterns of adverse effects that are very similar to those of combined oral contraceptives, with the exception of bleeding disturbances.
- In settings where postmarketing surveillance studies were carried out, Norplant proved to be a safe, well-tolerated, and highly effective contraceptive method.

Presentation 2
DATA AND ANALYSIS FROM POPULATION COUNCIL STUDIES
Irving Sivin
Center for Biomedical Research
Population Council

Background

Between 1990 and 1996, the Population Council conducted a series of studies to assess the health of women during use of either Norplant or what has been popularly referred to as "Norplant 2," now referred to as the LNG ROD or, outside the United States, Jadelle. The latter is an implant consisting of two rods that slowly release their levonorgestrel contents over an approved duration of efficacy of 3 years. The studies of this new formulation were undertaken to provide sufficient information to permit its registration, as well as to obtain additional information for revision of the efficacy labeling on Norplant. In the discussion that follows, "Norplant" refers to the slightly modified soft-tubing version approved by the Food and Drug Administration (FDA) for use in the United States.

Methodology

The studies involved a total population of 2,798 women in seven countries,[*] 43 percent of whom were from the United States.

- The first randomized study followed 199 women using an old version of the LNG ROD and 199 women using a new version of the LNG ROD. This study measured blood levels of drug, efficacy, and safety.
- The second randomized study involved 600 women using Norplant with the "soft" tubing and 600 women with the LNG ROD. It was mainly conducted outside the United States.

---

[*]Chile (2 sites), Dominican Republic, Egypt, Finland, Singapore, Thailand, United States (5 sites: University of Southern California, University of California at San Francisco, Robert Wood Johnson Research Institute, New York University, and Cornell University/ New York Medical Center).

- The third study, begun in 1990, was a non-randomized comparison study conducted mainly in the United States. This study trained clinic providers in the placement of Norplant in 600 women; the same clinics were subsequently provided with the LNG ROD for an additional 600 women. The studies included sexually active women aged 18 to 40, willing to give informed consent and to make regular visits. Women with histories of ectopic pregnancy and pelvic inflammatory disease since their last pregnancy were excluded. Women with evidence of depression, illness, and epilepsy were also excluded to ensure regular attendance. Follow-up consisted of multiple visits in Year 1 and semi-annual visits thereafter. Gynecological examinations were performed at each annual visit and, in many clinics, on a semi-annual basis.

Findings

The decision was made to analyze the three sets of studies collectively as "data on levonogestrel-releasing implants," because both Norplant and the LNG ROD were found to have similar hormonal release rates. The amount of levonogestrel released from Norplant was measured at approximately 70 milligrams over 5 years. Release rates for the LNG ROD were essentially identical; while, initially, there is a high daily release, at 200 days that rate decreases to about 50 micrograms per day and then slowly continues to decrease to about 25 micrograms per day.

Pregnancy and Continuation Rates

The two formulations are also identical in performance with regard to pregnancy and medical reasons for discontinuation:

- Gross pregnancy rates for both Norplant and the LNG ROD were identical at 0.4 per 100 woman-years at the end of 5 years in a randomized study overseas.
- For all studies taken together, for both formulations, the gross cumulative pregnancy rate at the end of 5 years was 1.0 per 100 woman-years, with a rate for the fifth year of 0.8 per 100.
- For the LNG ROD, the cumulative pregnancy rate at the end of 5 years was 1.2 per 100 woman-years, indistinguishable from that of Norplant.
- For the U.S. components of the study sample, the cumulative pregnancy rate for Norplant was 1.3 per 100 woman-years; for the LNG ROD, it was 0.7 per 100, again statistically indistinguishable and both highly effective.

As for ectopic pregnancies, in 9,300 woman-years over the course of the studies, there were two ectopic pregnancies, a rate of 0.22 per 1,000 woman-years.

There were no observable differences in discontinuation rates between the two formulations. The 1-year continuation rate for the studies as a group was over 90 out of 100 original adopters; at the end of 3 years, it was 70 per 100. Five-year continuation rates, for Norplant and for the LNG ROD, of Norplant II illustrate no significant differences; both methods had a 5-year continuation rate of over 50 per 100.

Reasons for Discontinuation

The principal reason for discontinuation of both versions of the implant was change in menstrual patterns, most importantly prolonged or irregular menstrual flow or increased bleeding. Approximately 9 to 10 percent of women using either method had terminated by the end of 2 years as a result of one or more of these problems. Table A-1 lists, for the group of studies as a whole, the conditions reported (limited to those experienced by more than 1 percent of the sample), the associated time points, and the percentages of women discontinuing implant use for those reasons.

TABLE A-1 Gross Cumulative Discontinuation Rates per 100, all 1990–1996 Population Council Norplant Studies

General Reason	Percentage *Terminated* for General Condition, 1 year	Percentage *Terminated* for General Condition, 5 years
Menstrual problems	4	20
Other medical problems	4	20
Planning pregnancy	1	20

For Individual Conditions	Percentage *Ever with* Condition		Percentage *Terminated* for Condition, 5 years
	1 year	5 years	
All Studies			
Vaginal discharge	9	28	0
Headache	16	28	3
Pelvic pain	9	22	<1
Weight increase	5	18	3
Acne	7	12	1
Mood change	3	5	1
Non-psychotic depression	1	3	<1
Alopecia (hair loss)	2	4	<1
U.S. Studies			
Vaginal discharge	10	25	0
Headache	15	25	2
Pelvic pain	10	23	<1
Weight increase	10	22	4
Acne	14	21	<1
Mood change	7	11	2
Non-psychotic depression	1	4	<1
Alopecia	5	9	<1

Removal Difficulties

Of 349 Norplant removals and 388 LNG ROD removals, 2.6 percent produced a complication, and that percentage was the same for both methods. The most common complications from the use of the LNG ROD resulted from unduly deep placement and multiple or excessively long incisions, each experienced by 1.3 percent of all women using that method. With Norplant, deep placement and bruising were the most frequent difficulties. Other complications such as broken capsules or rods did not produce adverse events. Not surprisingly, the LNG ROD produces fewer removal complications than Norplant and, because it consists of two rather than six elements, requires half the removal time. Even though removal times in the United States were longer than those in the other countries studied—in part because one of the five U.S. clinic sites (University of California at San Francisco) used the more time-consuming "pop-out" method and affected the overall average—removal times for the LNG ROD were shorter than those for Norplant.

Mortality and Hospitalization

For purposes of control, the Population Council data were compared to a 1995 U.S. hospital discharge survey and to data on high-income women collected in the United Kingdom by Martin Vessey in 1976; the comparisons were also controlled for age since the Vessey study included only women aged 25 and over. Mortality for the age groups represented is expected to be approximately 7 per 10,000. The mortality results per 10,000 woman-years of observation for each of these studies were as follows:

- Population Council studies, overall (9,300 woman-years): 1.1
- Population Council studies, U.S. sites (3,400 woman-years): 0.0
- Population Council studies, overall, women >25 (7,400 woman-years): 1.3;
- Population Council studies, U.S. sites, women >25 (2,600 woman-years): 0.0; and
- Vessey study (women aged >25):
  — oral contraceptives (31,076 woman-years): 4.8,
  — diaphragm (14,730 woman-years): 4.7, and
  — IUD (10,014 woman-years): 2.0.

The single death that occurred during the 5-year course of the Population Council studies was the result of an automobile accident in Bangkok, Thailand. In other words, the mortality rate at 5 years after initiating levonorgestrel implant use was well below the expected rate.

Hospitalization rates per 1,000 woman-years of observation were as follows:

- Population Council studies, overall: 20.7;
- Population Council studies, U.S. sites: 29.9;
- Population Council studies, overall, women >25: 19.7;
- Population Council studies, U.S. sites, women >25: 25.0; and
- Vessey study:
  - oral contraceptives: 50.9,
  - diaphragm: 54.0, and
  - IUD: 57.7.

The U.S. hospital discharge survey found a hospitalization rate for women aged 15 to 44 of 130,000 to 140,000 per 1000 woman-years depending on survey year; when pregnancy-related hospitalizations are extracted, that rate falls to approximately 62 per 1,000. The rate of 20.7 for the Population Council implant studies as a whole is still notably lower. It is also lower than all hospitalization rates found in the Vessey studies. There is no body system in which implants have elevated hospitalization rates compared with the U.S. hospital discharge survey or Vessey's studies.

Conclusions

- Norplant and the LNG ROD provide essentially identical drug release and clinical performance through 3 to 5 years of use.
- The cumulative pregnancy rates through 5 years of use are approximately 1 to 1.5 per 100, comparable to those associated with sterilization or the levonogestrel-releasing IUD.
- Menstrual and medical complaints associated with the use of these implants are frequent and require counseling before and during use, yet women continue to use the implants at rates higher than almost all other reversible methods of contraception.
- Removal is markedly faster with the LNG ROD, but training in placement and removal is still required and maintenance of skills essential. Correct insertion is the prerequisite to easy removal.
- Severe adverse events are uncommon among implant users. Death rates have been zero in the United States in over 3,000 women years and 1.1 per 10,000 woman-years of observation for the 1990–1996 Population Council studies overall. Hospitalization rates among users in the U.S. studies have been substantially below rates for all U.S. women aged 15 to 44.
- Low pregnancy rates, high continuation rates, and the safety profiles indicate that Norplant and the LNG ROD are a reasonable contraceptive choice for American and non-American women of reproductive age.

Presentation 3
BIOCOMPATIBILITY AND MEDICAL APPLICATIONS OF SILICONE-BASED MATERIALS: REVIEW OF PERTINENT FINDINGS
Noel Rose, M.D., Ph.D.
The Johns Hopkins University

Background

The main issues surrounding silicone concern silicone gel-filled breast implants. Despite earlier contentions that implicated these implants in autoimmune diseases, more recent epidemiological studies refute this association. However, this debate did stimulate research on possible immunological effects deriving from a wider range of silicone implants.

Related research at the Rochester General Hospital produced findings in a rat model that silicone gel can act as an adjuvant, which is most simply described as a substance with the ability to enhance the immune response to a foreign or self-antigen. Despite the fact that millions of individuals have safely received adjuvants over the past 70 years as components of standard childhood vaccines, the Rochester report evoked concern. The concern was based on misunderstanding of what happens when adjuvants couple with self-antigen to produce, in laboratory models, autoimmune disease, in which pathology results from a misguided or misdirected immune response deleterious to the host. In response to that understanding, the Rochester study was reevaluated so as to confirm, or not, the contention that silicone gel can, in fact, serve as an adjuvant and, further, to see whether silicone elastomer of the type used in Norplant might have adjuvant properties.[*]

Methodology

Both rats and mice were used in these experiments. A standard adjuvant (Freund's) was used as the positive control and the silicone oil/gel mixture used in the Rochester study was the experimental material. All these materials were combined with a foreign substance, bovine serum albumen (BSA), to see whether there was any adjuvant effect. The procedure called for bleeding the rats and mice from the heart at regular intervals, carrying out tests to see how much antibody to BSA was present in the serum, and then sacrificing the animal at the end of the experiment and examining the implant sites.

In a second experiment, rats were injected with BSA mixed with particles of silicone elastomer of the type used in Norplant. Both large and small particles were used to reproduce the possible effects for breaking up over the life span of an

---

[*] JO Naim, RJ Lanzafame, and CJ Van Oss. The effect of silicone-gel on the immune response. *Journal of Biomaterial Science-Polymer Edition* 7(2);123–132, 1995.

implant in the body. At the end of the experiment, the rats were sacrificed, their serum tested for antibody to BSA, and the injection sites examined histologically for evidence of inflammation.

A third experiment was performed to determine if the antigen (BSA) must be carefully and extensively homogenized with the gel/oil combination before injection or whether the two ingredients could simply be mixed as would occur in the body.

Findings

The gel/oil combination was compared with Freund's adjuvant in its ability to potentiate the response to a foreign substance (BSA); the two adjuvants proved to be equivalent. These results confirmed the findings of the Rochester group and extended them to another species, the mouse. In contrast to the results of the first experiment, neither the large nor the small particles of the silicone elastomer had any adjuvant effect when mixed with BSA. The elastomer particles did produce a marked local inflammatory response consisting mostly of macrophages and lymphocytes. Thus, the presence of an inflammatory response does not entail adjuvant activity. Both the gel/oil and elastomer particles produced an inflammatory effect, but only the gel/oil had any adjuvant effect. Furthermore, the only way of showing the adjuvant effect of the gel/oil is to homogenize it outside the body with a foreign material, BSA. Simply mixing antigen with gel/oil does not produce an adjuvant effect. Neither the large nor the small particles of the silicone elastomer potentiated antibody response in the rat model. Thus, any silicone elastomer particulates that might come off the Norplant implant would, similarly, have no adjuvant effect even though both large and small particles can incite a respectable inflammatory response.

Conclusions

These experiments indicate that there is no risk of developing autoimmune disease associated with implants of silicone elastomer.

Presentation 4
BIOCOMPATIBILITY AND MEDICAL APPLICATIONS OF SILICONE-BASED MATERIALS: REVIEW OF PERTINENT FINDINGS
James M. Anderson, M.D., Ph.D.
Case Western Reserve University

Background

This presentation summarizes what is known about those aspects of the silicone-based materials used in contraceptive implants that would permit conclusions about any possible relationships between those materials and human systemic effects. It reports on studies of the biocompatibility, or biological response testing, of the silicone rubber that is a component of the Norplant implant system, and the inherent characteristics of that biomaterial.

Findings

Composition

Norplant is an exceptionally small implant, consisting of six tubes with a volume just above 1 cubic centimeter and a surface area of 18 square centimeters. It is composed of a medical-grade elastomer, the tube material itself, and a medical-grade adhesive. The formulation is to take this dimethylmethylvinylsiloxane, dimethylvinyl terminated material, a polymer, and incorporate it with a short-chain material called dimethylsiloxane, which is hydroxy terminated in the presence of amorphous silica and then reacted at elevated temperatures with a free-radical-producing material, which comes from benzoyl peroxide. Once extruded and cured, the tube is filled and then sealed with a medical-grade adhesive. Two reactive materials ultimately crosslink the silica together with the polymer chain. In the prepolymer are types of chemical groups which, in the presence of the free radical, can provide for crosslinking as well as chain extensions, since this occurs at the end of the chain.

Because of the highly crosslinked structures created with the free radicals and extrusion, silicone rubbers are some of the most difficult materials to characterize chemically. The adhesive is very similar; it contains hydroxy-terminated materials, highly reactive when they react with small silane molecules called methyltriaceytoxysilane. When reacted together, this hydroxyl group will react with an aceytoxy group and bind two silicones through an oxygen group, releasing acetic acid. There is a small bit of a plasticizer present, but when all these things react together, the result is a cured silicone medical adhesive which plugs the tubes.

The filler material is not crystalline silica but amorphous silica that is not associated, as is crystalline silica, with pathological problems, and is added to enhance the mechanical properties of the material. It is treated with a silazane type of material that allows the silica particle to react directly with the polymer chain that is formed, which in turn assists in holding this particle within the network structure.

Although concerns have been raised about silica rubbing off other silicone implants, recent studies by Ratner[*] have shown that the surface properties of filled silicone elastomers do not include potential for abrasion. Ratner took both silica-filled and silica-free polydimethylsiloxane (PDMS) and used both amorphous and

---

[*] BD Ratner et al., *1994 Annual Meeting Transactions of the Society for Biomaterials*. Vol. XVII, p. 22, 1994.

crystalline silica. These were then treated with abrasion, enzymes, and hydrogen peroxide. Using very sensitive mass spectrometry techniques that sample only the outer 20 to 80 angstroms (or, with SIMS, 10 to 15 angstroms), the Ratner studies detected no silica in the outermost surface area. Because these polymers have the PDMS outer coating, it is that silicone polymer, not amorphous silica, that is present at the surface.

Inflammatory Wound Healing Reaction and Blood Protein Absorption

Experience with silicone rubber and PDMS over the past decade was also studied, including *in vitro* studies with blood protein absorption and macrophage activation with cytokine release, as well as *in vivo* studies of inflammatory response and resolution, and fibrous capsule formation.

As with any implant, when Norplant is implanted, it becomes coated with blood protein. The cells that then interact in the inflammatory and wound healing response encounter a protein-coated material. There seems to be no difference in materials when they are coated with the blood protein. An illustration: A silicone rubber circulating in a blood pump system up to 180 minutes—fibrinogen, IGG, albumen, fibronectin, factor 12 in the coagulation system, factor VIII—are all comparable. Most protein absorption occurs within the first 5 minutes, all of it within 15 minutes. There has been some recent literature that the IGG is an antipolymer antibody. However, IGG's binding to the polymer surface is not new; when a foreign material is inserted, blood proteins absorb and IGG, along with complement, adheres to those surfaces.

The activation of human monocyte cultures and the release of cytokines which can cause subsequent and possibly systemic events were also studied. Interleukin-1 coming from monocytes/macrophages in zones of inflammation has been linked to fever production, a correlation that generally leads to the belief that it causes fever when it systemically circulates and reaches the brain. In PDMS, however, different cytokines are seen released from a cell culture and PDMS with no protein is noticeably below the polystyrene control, as are the IL-6 and the tumor necrosis factor.

The activation of the macrophages is reduced when the silicone rubber is precoated with protein, for example, IGG coated onto the silicone rubber, a general phenomenon in which the blood protein appears to reduce the activation of those cells on the surface. Activity was measured by bioassay and concentration was measured by a radio immunoassay for interleukin-1, and there was no protein absorption. PDMS is of the same order as biomer, a polyurethane used in catheters; dacron, which is used in many applications; and polyethylene, which is also used in catheters as well as in hip and knee implants.

Bioresponsiveness and early inflammatory response were tested by putting PDMS into a cage of stainless steel mesh, and the resolution of inflammatory response was then monitored over a 21-day period. Not only did the numbers at any given time period prove to be comparable between the polymers, but the decrease in inflammatory cells out to day 21 was also comparable. Monocytes and interleukin-1 activity were also monitored over that same 21-day time period. While PDMS appeared to show an increase in interleukin-1 activity, it dropped off in the same way as the polyethylene control and showed decreased activation compared to the empty-cage control. The same pattern was observed in an *in vitro/in vivo* comparison for interleukin-1 activity released from human monocytes in culture vis-à-vis the monocytes from rat exudates in the cage.

Any material that is implanted, in effect, creates an injury which then produces an inflammatory response. Monocytes that circulate in the bloodstream, in addition to polymorphonuclear leukocytes, are the principal defense team that migrates into those tissues to combat the invader. Polymorphonuclear leukocytes have a very short lifetime, but monocytes differentiate in the macrophages which then migrate onto the surface of the material. A fibrous capsule develops around the implant and then, at the surface, there is a one- to two-cell layer of macrophages and their fusion product, called giant cells or foreign-body giant cells. Macrophages and their fusion product have been present at implants that have been in individuals for two to three decades, so that this is a persistent response present at all biomaterial or medical device prosthetic interfaces with tissue.

The macrophages, releasing interleukin-1, then fuse together so that they have multinucleated giant cells. An early fibrous capsule containing numerous fibroblasts forms. Then, as the wound heals, usually within 3 to 4 weeks, the capsule condenses and becomes acellular, and some of the vascularity present in the early fibrous capsule may actually be lost. With an implant like Norplant, the capsule is expected to be well healed and, within 3 to 4 weeks, to become a relatively acellular capsule without many capillaries so that the position of the implant stabilizes. The foreign body reaction, consisting of macrophages and foreign body giant cells at the interface, is also expected to become quiescent and not cause many problems, as indeed it has not. Quantitative measurement of fibrous capsules in rats, looking at various types of materials, shows that at 4 weeks reactions to PDMS are considerably less than those associated with dacron, polyethylene, or expanded polytetrafluoroethylene.

In sum, using both *in vitro* and *in vivo* methods, silicone rubber, or silica-free PDMS, displayed responses that were similar or better than those biomaterials. Although it is believed that the acellular fibrous capsule that forms over the implant does not affect the pharmacokinetics of the drug because it is avascular, this depends on the solubility parameters of the drug used. For instance, in a classic example, published 30 years ago, silicone rubber was used; tested in humans, the capsule proved to have become saturated because the drug had crystallized. The fibrous capsule may have played a role in controlling release of the drug, or may simply have acted as another barrier, with the drug dissolving out of the fibrous capsule and then into systemic circulation.

Conclusions

Studies conducted by researchers at Case Western Reserve on the biocompatibility, or biological response testing, of silicone rubber and its inherent characteristics as a component of Norplant, have led to the conclusion that it is not immune system reaction but polymer supply and availability of biomaterials that constitute the greatest challenge to the contraceptive industry. Years of tort litigation about silicone rubber used in the production of medical devices have culminated in what is now a crisis in the availability of biomaterials for many implant technologies. When the major chemical companies finally and totally discontinue production and sales of silicone rubber and related products, the small quantities of silicone materials that are needed for contraceptive implants will no longer be available. Some of the "mirror image" silicone rubbers now being tested by companies are inadequate in the chemical properties that, for a 5-year implant like Norplant, are integral to its success since it is the maintenance of the integrity of the shell that sustains its perfusion properties. Reform of tort laws concerning silicone should continue to include provisions for holding accountable the company producing a given device; the problem of supply stems from the fear that accountability is not limited to that company alone, but often extends to the suppliers of raw materials.

Presentation 5
VAGINAL HIV/SIV TRANSMISSION: MONKEY SIV DATA
Preston A. Marx, Ph.D.
Aaron Diamond AIDS Research Center

Background

A rhesus macaque monkey model was developed to investigate progesterone's effect on vaginal simian immunodeficiency virus (SIV) transmission. As estrogen and progesterone influence the fitness of the vaginal epithelium, the hypothesis was that progesterone will diminish the vaginal barrier and increase vaginal transmission of SIV. The model was initially developed to get a clearer understanding of the early pathogenesis of SIV transmission. During these experiments, cell-free SIV was inserted into the vagina without trauma, since trauma was unnecessary as the virus transmits across intact vaginal epithelium.

One of the first findings from these studies was that the intact vaginal epithelium was a strong barrier to infection. Intravenous transmission of SIV proves to be the most sensitive way to introduce an HIV-like virus into a monkey or HIV into a human. Intravenously, the virus simply needs to come in contact with a susceptible lymphoid cell to initiate infection; it has very few barriers to cross. The vaginal mucosa therefore required 1,000 times more virus to elicit an infection and even at this increased dose, infection in every animal is not guaranteed.

Cell-free virus transmission contrasts markedly to cell-associated virus transmission. Evidence of the difference in amount of virus that is required to establish infection intravenously compared to vaginally does not indicate that cell-associated transmission cannot happen in this model, only that it is more difficult.

The speed of progression of disease constitutes the major difference between the SIV macaque model and human beings: Disease develops up to three times faster in the SIV macaque model than in a human being infected with HIV. Following challenge with SIV, animals are characterized in several ways. Rapid progressors are those not producing antibody response, and therefore showing relatively continuous growth in viral load, as is the case in human beings. Progressors display antibody response and are capable of suppressing virus. Slow-progressors and non-progressors are also identifiable. Research has been conducted to study this process and the difference between rapid progressors and progressors. Almost certainly a fundamental mechanism exists in the way the virus activates the T cells, causing them to become susceptible.

Langerhans and dendritic cells located in the epithelium and mucosa are susceptible to HIV and SIV infection. In fact, studies have been done from cadaver material in human beings and in monkeys that indicate that these cells tend to migrate out and become infected. The function of the Langerhans cell is to sample the vaginal lumen, pick up foreign antigens, and carry them back to the nearest lymph node. This mechanism allows HIV and SIV to infiltrate the body rapidly. Looking at the Langerhans cells, dendritic cells, the vaginal lumen, and epithelium, using *in situ* polymerase chain reaction (PCR), infection and trafficking of dendritic cells can be seen by Day 2. So, the infection begins quite early and in as little as three days or less enters the immune system.

These initial findings serve as the basis for this model and its usefulness in addressing the question of progesterone's effect on the transmission of SIV.

Methodology

Initially, placebo implants and progesterone implants were inserted into 28 animals, with 10 placebo animals and 18 progesterone-implanted animals used to ensure a chance of statistically significant results. The vaginal challenge was done at 4 to 5 days after implant insertion, using a virus titer to infect less than 10 percent of the animals. This protocol was intentionally designed to show an increase in the rate of infection. The placebo group of animals was challenged during the follicular phase, when the vaginal epithelium is its thickest. The test group with the progesterone implants was challenged 4 to 5 days after the second implant. Weekly virus counts, antibody assays, PCR, and virus load determinants by branch DNA were performed in both groups. Several lymph node biopsies were taken. These animals were watched for several months for determination of disease status.

Following the first set of results, a second experiment using six animals was performed, the purpose of which was to monitor virus action within the first week post-implantation. Three animals received placebo implants and three received progesterone implants. This set of animals was euthanized within 3 days of exposure and vaginal epithelium was analyzed.

Findings

One animal from the placebo group and 14 of the 18 animals in the progesterone group became infected with SIV. Several of these animals progressed quite rapidly to disease, which is unusual given such a low virus dose.

The second experiment of six animals served as a model to show the first target cells. All three of the placebo animals remained negative. In the progesterone group, virus was recoverable from two of the animals, one harboring virus in the blood, plasma, and iliac lymph node, and the other in the spleen and iliac node. The third animal remained negative.

The vaginal epithelium was graded based on a system developed at Harvard Medical School. Grades of 1 to 3 were assigned to epithelium based on cell number thickness. The epithelium appeared to be much thinner when progesterone was present.

Conclusions

The thick versus thin hypothesis is that a thick epithelium will allow less virus through and a thin vaginal epithelium is less likely to provide protection and will allow more virus to come through. Transmission may occur through breaks, infected cells or, if cell-free virus, infection of a dendritic cell which then migrates to the draining nodes. The hypothesis is that a thick epithelium will allow less virus through.

Other effects of progesterone warrant attention. There may be an influx of target cells into the epithelium, the cervix, and the lumen, and if the progesterone causes more target cells to be available, this could play a role in enhanced transmission and in immune changes in the host, including perhaps some immune suppression. The effect on the physiology of the host cell receptors, where viral growth and replication are possible, also requires further analysis. Estrogen could also have effects, since it does have effects on the immune system and changes in target cells.

The question of whether or not changes in the estrogen and progesterone levels affect vaginal transmission has been addressed only preliminarily. One experiment found that vaginal epithelium, thinned by progesterone, enhanced transmission. The rhesus model should be helpful as a mechanism to gain insight into how the natural changes in the estrogen and progesterone levels before and after ovulation affect susceptibility to infection, and to determine if estrogen plays a protective role by thickening the vaginal epithelium. The model might also serve as a useful model for menopause, to look at the effect of vaginal transmission of viral infection in an absence of hormones.

Presentation 6
VAGINAL HIV/SIV TRANSMISSION: HUMAN EPIDEMIOLOGICAL DATA
Willard Cates, Jr., M.D., M.P.H.
Family Health International

Background and Methodology

In a recent evaluation, Family Health International (FHI) reviewed the role contraception plays in a range of factors affecting sexual transmission of human immunodeficiency virus (HIV). Our basic knowledge includes a general understanding that the most powerful predictor of HIV transmission is the stage of infection during which sexual contact occurs, with probability of transmission highest during late-stage infection, during very early-stage infection when viral load is highest, and/or concurrent with the presence of other sexually transmitted diseases (STDs) of the type that are ulcerative or productive of discharge.

Important among the elements of the review was an examination of relationships, either protective or facilitative, between hormonal contraceptives and HIV transmission. Because no data are available from Level 1 studies—that is, randomized controlled trials—the review depended on epidemiologically based data from Level 2–3 studies—that is, well-controlled cohort studies. Of approximately 25 observational studies which collected data on HIV transmission and oral contraception, the majority were cross-sectional, which meant that no conclusions could be drawn about direction of causality. Only 9 of the studies were of Level 2 quality.

Findings

The range of association, in a variety of populations for combined oral contraceptives containing both estrogens and progestins, extended from a protective effect of 0.6 to a harmful effect of 4.5; no conclusions can be drawn from such a range. Since a measure of relative risk equal to 1 means no effect, any measure less than 1 is considered protective, and any measure greater than 1 indicates a harmful association. In studies where the quality of evidence is weaker, relative risks below 2 may be confounded by many biases, including risk of sexual exposure, contextual and biological factors affecting transmission, and behavioral variables that may mask biological impact.

As for the relationship between implanted hormones and HIV transmission, no studies with large enough populations to permit solid, directly attributable conclusions have been conducted. However, the injectable hormone Depo-Provera has been used as a contraceptive progestin in human beings in four Level 2 studies. In two of those, the relative risks straddle 1; in the remaining two, one in Thailand and one in Kenya, the relative risks are 1.9 and 3.4, respectively. Again, conclusions are confounded by the biases of observational studies.

At a June 1996 consensus panel meeting at the National Institute of Child Health and Human Development, a systematic effort was made to draw some tentative conclusions about etiology from the available observational studies. No causal inferences were possible because: (1) consistency among the studies is poor; (2) the strength of association is quite small; (3) few of the studies reviewed are adequately powered; (4) prospective data are limited; (5) most of the studies are cross-sectional and thus unable to demonstrate whether the contraceptive use or the HIV prevalence being measured occurred first; and (6) a relative risk below 2 in an observational study can be affected by numerous types of bias.

Confounding is also a problem inherent in observational studies, and perhaps especially so in this case, given the multiplicity of possible factors that can contribute to sexual transmission of infection. In addition to stage of infection and concurrent STD, these include sexual practices, circumcision (male or female), cervical ectopy, genetic factors, immunological factors, and contraceptive method. To this already large and complex group must be added a subset of factors that are likely to be implicated in the relationship between hormones and HIV transmission: menstrual patterns, vaginal immunology, and the role of and effects on vaginal epithelium and cervical mucus.

The consensus panel concluded that until better human studies become available, the most prudent path will be to reorder clinical management priorities for counselling high-risk clients. The first priority for these clients is to ensure protection from sexually transmitted infections (i.e., through regular condom use and other risk-reduction strategies); optimal protection against conception (i.e., through implant use) becomes second priority. Workshop participants noted that human studies including vaginal biopsies are also being developed and commented that the potential for doing randomized studies in human populations will be both ethically and practically challenging.

Conclusions

Following this presentation was a discussion about the need for well-designed human studies. The question arose as to whether better designed observational studies might be able to provide the necessary data, given questions about the ethics and feasibility of trials among condom users that would involve randomization to use of a hormonal birth control method or placebo. The case was made that ethics and feasibility would both reside in the order in which recruitment to such a study occurred. Individuals who had first chosen condoms as their primary method of contraception could then be recruited, in which case assignment to additional use of a hormonal method or placebo would not put them at risk of disease transmission or undue risk of conception. The suggestion was made that community-based informed consent processes would be particularly appropriate to such studies. The question arose about the extent to which such a sample would be representative of the general population.

Another ethical question had to do with risk/benefit issues. A basic ethical tenet of research is that if a group in a randomized controlled trial would be worse off than without the study, then the study becomes unethical by definition. If the group would be better off than otherwise, then randomization becomes justified. However, in trials involving contraception and protection against infection, the matter becomes more complex and the counseling and informed consent processes require special and careful thought.

Presentation 7
DATA AND ANALYSIS FROM THE
1995 NATIONAL SURVEY OF FAMILY GROWTH
Jacqueline E. Darroch, Ph.D.
The Alan Guttmacher Institute

Background

The National Survey of Family Growth (NSFG) is the most comprehensive source of information available on pregnancy and contraceptive use among reproductive-age women in the United States. Conducted by the National Center for Health Statistics, it is a federally funded series of household surveys carried out in 1973, 1976, 1982, 1988, and, most recently, 1995. Analysis of the 1995 data is in various stages of completion but enough information was available to inform this workshop. The 1995 NSFG surveyed a randomized, nationally representative sample of 10,847 women between the ages of 15 and 44, and gathered information about sexual behavior, contraceptive use, pregnancy, and infertility.

Findings

The NSFG found that just 1 percent of the women in the sample—104 of the 10,847 women surveyed—were using Norplant, a proportion consistent with that found in the 1996 Ortho Birth Control Study. Women who had ever used the implant totaled 2 percent.

Despite the constraints imposed on analysis by the small number of Norplant users, the NSFG data do permit additional insights into who those users are. Multivariate analysis revealed that Norplant use was importantly affected by age, Medicaid coverage, parity, and geography, with age the most strongly associated factor. Most women in the NSFG sample who were currently using Norplant were under age 30. Women aged 20–24 were the largest group of users, representing 4 percent of all women using reversible contraceptive methods and a little under 4 percent of all women contracepting. Women aged 15–19 were proportionally the next largest group, followed by women aged 25–29. Women over age 30 accounted for progressively smaller proportions of Norplant users.

Most Norplant users have had one child, often at an early age, and these younger contraceptors, especially those in their early 20s, are much more likely to use Norplant than women of the same age who are not on Medicaid. Patterns of method continuation suggest that these women are using Norplant primarily for birth spacing. The rate of initial Norplant use then begins to decrease with greater parity, as women with two or more children turn to sterilization, although there is some bimodal distribution as more older women of higher parity adopt Norplant as a long-term, reversible alternative to tubal ligation.

Norplant use was also affected by geography. Norplant use is substantially lower in the northeastern portion of the United States than in the midwestern, southern, and western regions of the country, with the western region showing the highest utilization. These differences may have to do with variations in service provision, but this remains to be explored.

Factors determined not to have independent predictive importance for Norplant use were education, marital status, race, ethnicity, poverty, or residence (metropolitan/nonmetropolitan, central city/suburban). Despite small differences across these variables, none proved significant when controlled for age, parity, Medicaid status, and region.

Conclusions

Overall, the small number of Norplant users limits this data set as a tool for further analysis, and underscores the importance of performing other types of targeted clinic studies with samples large enough to allow more generalized understandings about this method and its use. The NSFG found that at least one-third of women using Norplant obtained it from a clinic, so that knowledge about this subpopulation will continue to be critical.

Presentation 8
UTILIZATION DATA
Debra Kalmuss, Ph.D., *and*
Andrew R. Davidson, Ph.D., M.B.A.
Columbia University[*]

Background

The factors surrounding women's decisions to continue or discontinue Norplant as a method of contraception were highlighted in a recently completed 5-

---

[*]Kalmuss D, and A Davidson. *Norplant Discontinuation among Low-Income Women.* Supported by the National Institute of Child Health and Human Development/NIH and the Henry J. Kaiser Family Foundation.

year, multicenter study supported by the National Institute of Child Health and Development and the Henry J. Kaiser Family Foundation. The study was designed to, first, identify factors influencing initial selection of a contraceptive method; second, obtain rates and determinants of Norplant discontinuation; and, third, discover whether there were either provider or cost barriers to implant removal. The study was modified during its course to incorporate questions about the effects of the negative media coverage of Norplant that began in March 1994.

Methodology

Patients were recruited in three hospital-based clinic sites: New York City (Presbyterian), Pittsburgh (Magee-Women's), and Dallas (Parkland). The clienteles of these clinics and, therefore, of the study samples were primarily young, low-income, minority women with active fertility histories, recruited after having selected a method of contraception but prior to having received it, in order to assess expectations prior to experience with the method. Forty percent of these women had had one unintended pregnancy and 30 percent had had two or more such pregnancies. Almost 40 percent had one live birth, another 38 percent had two, and 15 percent had more than two live births. Sixty-one percent of the sample had their first birth during their teenage years and over one-third had had that first birth at age 17 or younger. Total sample size was 2,003 and consisted of 491 women who had chosen Depo-Provera, 314 who had chosen oral contraceptives, 288 who had chosen tubal ligation, and 910 who had chosen Norplant, with the last group oversampled to permit acquisition of significant data on rates and determinants of discontinuation. Norplant selectors were interviewed at baseline and followed up at 6 months post-insertion and then either at time of removal of the implant or at 2 years post-insertion, whichever came first. Women who selected either the pill or sterilization were interviewed only at baseline and only about initial method choice, and not followed after that first interview. Women who selected Depo-Provera were interviewed at baseline and followed up at 12 months post-initiation for insights into their experiences and comparative data on method discontinuation. Rates of follow-up were high: 90 percent of women who had selected Norplant were followed for at least one time point and 85 percent of the women who had selected Depo-Provera were re-interviewed at 12 months.

Findings and Conclusions

Sample Characteristics

Mean age of the study sample was 22. Two-thirds had annual household incomes under $10,000, 90 percent under $20,000. Sixty-one percent were Hispanic, 23 percent African American, and 16 percent white.

Continuation and Discontinuation

During the first 12 months of use, rates of Norplant discontinuation increased in linear fashion with no sharp breaks in the line. At the 6-month time point, 8 percent had discontinued use; at 12 months, the cumulative discontinuation rate was 23 percent. In the group of women who had selected Depo-Provera, the 12-month discontinuation rate was 55 percent; 50 percent of all discontinuers stopped after their first injection.

These rates surprised family planning providers, who appear to share the perception that Depo-Provera is far more popular than Norplant. However, this perception may be an artifact of the different nature of clinic re-visits associated with these methods. For Norplant, a clinic visit is required for discontinuation but not for continuation. For Depo-Provera, the situation is reversed. As such, providers are seeing "happy" Depo-Provera users and "unhappy" Norplant users which, in turn, biases provider conclusions about continuation rates and may well affect their attitudes when counseling clients about prospective method use.

Logistic regression analysis indicated the following predictors of early Norplant discontinuation (i.e., within the first 6 months of use): dissatisfaction with prior contraceptive methods, a partner who wants a child within the next two years, perceived pressure from a health care provider to initiate Norplant use, exposure to negative media coverage, and the number of implant side effects. Women's social and demographic characteristics, Medicaid status, and motivation to avoid an unplanned pregnancy were not significantly related to early removal. Preliminary analysis of the determinants of 2-year discontinuation point to the importance of two additional determinants, the woman's fertility desires and whether her Norplant side effects were worse than she expected.

The study also examined the outcomes of discontinuation among Depo-Provera users. Women who discontinue Depo-Provera are at very high risk for unintended pregnancy, with a rate of unintended pregnancy of 17 percent at 6 months after discontinuation and, at 9 months, 20 percent. Those rates among teenagers are especially high. Follow-up analysis of those rates for women discontinuing Norplant use is still in progress.

Media Effects

Negative media coverage beginning in the early spring of 1994 produced a dramatic effect on implant insertions.[*] In 1991, 1992, and 1993 insertions had grown steadily, averaging over 100 per month in large hospital-based family planning programs. Following critical media events beginning in March 1994, insertions fell to fewer than 10 per month. Although Depo-Provera, which appeared on the U.S. market in 1993, is thought to have taken some of the

---

[*] See "Effects of Media Coverage and Litigation on Norplant Use" (p. 21) and Figure 2-1 (p. 22).

Norplant market, it is unlikely to have precipitated the sudden, very large drop in insertions that began in the second quarter of 1994. Implant removals also rose during this period, an increase that remains substantial even after the numbers are adjusted for women identified as at risk for removal.

Norplant and Coercion

This study explored whether low-income women perceived that providers were steering them onto Norplant. Of the 2,000 women interviewed, only 3 said that they felt any pressure from a health care provider to use Norplant. The absence of steering was further reflected in women's responses to a question probing why they had chosen Norplant. Only 4 women cited health care provider influence as a reason for their choice. Finally, the data show that the process of obtaining Norplant runs counter to the claim of coercion. Norplant adopters had to make significantly more clinic visits to obtain their method than did women seeking oral contraceptives. In addition, women rated the process of obtaining Norplant as more difficult than that for the pill.

The study also examined whether provider- and cost-based barriers impeded access to Norplant removal. Preliminary analyses suggest a mixed picture with regard to removal barriers. On the one hand, most women reported no barriers to removal. On the other hand, a sizable minority of women experienced or anticipated one or more provider- or cost-based barriers to Norplant removal, although women's anticipation of removal barriers far exceeded their actual experience of such barriers. These findings support the need for clearly stated policies of removal upon demand that are more effectively communicated to women considering the method.

Presentation 9
WOMEN'S EXPERIENCE WITH NORPLANT: A COMPARISON WITH DEPO-PROVERA AND ORAL CONTRACEPTIVES
Helen P. Koo, Ph.D.[*]
Research Triangle Institute

Background

This 4-year longitudinal study of contraceptive choice and use compared the experiences women had with Norplant, Depo-Provera, and the oral contraceptive

---

[*] Koo HP, JD Griffith, ME Nennstiel, WL Graves, RA Hatcher, and S Laurent. *Women's Experience with Norplant: A Comparison with Depo-Provera and Oral Contraceptives.* Research Triangle Institute, Emory University, and Carolinas Medical Center. Supported by the National Institute of Child Health and Human Development/NIH and the Henry J. Kaiser Family Foundation.

(OC) pill. The study focused on rates of, and reasons for, discontinuation, as well as women's assessments of their experiences. The study also was designed to study the choice of Norplant compared to other methods.

Methodology

Baseline data were collected from July 1993 to October 1994 at urban family planning and postpartum clinics, maternity wards, and ambulatory surgeries in Atlanta, Georgia, and Charlotte, North Carolina. The sample was a probability sample of African American and white women who were choosing a contraceptive method different from the one they had used in the preceding 3 months, with options including Norplant, Depo-Provera, oral contraceptives, condoms, or female sterilization. The baseline survey focused on factors affecting choice of the methods and expectations about them. A first follow-up survey was conducted by telephone between November 1994 and April 1996, and a second follow-up telephone survey between April 1996 and May 1997. The follow-up surveys took monthly histories of contraceptive use, pregnancies, and months with no sexual intercourse, and determined discontinuation over time, reasons for discontinuation, experiences with side effects, assessments of method used, switches to other methods and non-use, and reasons for switches. In addition, to gain insight into possible experiences with coercion, women who planned, considered, or had an implant removed were interviewed concerning perceptions of pressures from a provider to retain it.

To compare the probability of discontinuation over time of Norplant with that of Depo-Provera and the pill, hazards models were estimated, in which differences in characteristics of women selecting these methods were accounted for. These included the following baseline variables: age, postpartum status, number of planned and unplanned pregnancies, plans for more children, race, education of the person who raised the respondent, Medicaid status, enrollment in Aid to Families with Dependent Children (AFDC) or food stamps, number of problems encountered at the clinic, and study site. The hazards model for discontinuation from all causes also examined the effects of the severity of menstrual and nonmenstrual side effects (as determined in the first follow-up survey).

Findings

Sample Characteristics

Of the eligible population, 2,477 (86%) responded to the survey during baseline data collection which took place from July 1993 to October 1994; 1,840 women (86.7% of non-sterilized respondents) participated in the first follow-up telephone survey.

At the baseline, 330 women had chosen Norplant, 787 had chosen Depo-Provera, and 889 had chosen the pill. Of the women interviewed in the follow-up, some had changed method and analysis was adjusted to take these changes into account. Thus, final numbers used for analysis were 303 segments of use of Norplant, 879 of Depo-Provera, and 1,008 of the pill.

Taken as a whole, the sample shared a number of characteristics. Women at both sites tended to be young, African American, lower-income, and receiving some sort of public assistance. Most had had at least one pregnancy, half had two or more, and about 70 percent of all past pregnancies in the group as a whole had been unplanned. More than half of the sample wanted more children.

However, all of these characteristics differed significantly across methods. Norplant users tended to be slightly older than women using the pill or Depo-Provera, of higher parity and with more unplanned pregnancies, less likely to want more children, more likely to be receiving public assistance, and much more likely to be Medicaid clients. Pill users as a group had had the fewest pregnancies, including the fewest unplanned pregnancies, and fewer were postpartum. Pill users were also much more likely to want more children, and much less likely than Norplant and Depo-Provera users to be receiving AFDC or food stamps or to be on Medicaid. Depo-Provera users were younger as a group than either Norplant or pill users and more likely to be African American.

Continuation and Discontinuation

Women using Norplant were more likely to have experienced severe menstrual side effects than were women using either Depo-Provera or the pill. For each method, discontinuation was highest in women with severe menstrual side effects and, unsurprisingly, lowest for women with no side effects. Still, even for women with severe menstrual side effects, the 12-month discontinuation rate was by far the lowest for Norplant users. Similar results were found for severity of nonmenstrual side effects.

Nearly all Norplant and Depo-Provera users had experienced some menstrual or nonmenstrual side effects; fewer, but a substantial majority of pill users, had at least one. Women using Norplant were considerably more likely to experience longer periods, irregular cycles, heavier bleeding, and headaches than were women using the other two methods, although Depo-Provera users were the most likely of the three user groups to have problems with amenorrhea and weight gain. Norplant users also had a greater number of different side effects.

Nevertheless, the rate of discontinuation of Norplant by 12 months was just 15 percent and nearly all of this was due to side effects (either menstrual or nonmenstrual). The discontinuation rate due to side effects was more than twice that percentage for those using Depo-Provera or the pill. For all three methods, discontinuation due to nonmenstrual side effects was higher than was the case for menstrual side effects. Discontinuation by 12 months because of unintended pregnancy was negligible for Norplant and Depo-Provera. Discontinuation for reasons other than side effects or pregnancy was also negligible for Norplant but not for the other two methods. For both Depo-Provera and the pill, "forgetting" and "inconvenience" were important contributors to discontinuation.

As for user satisfaction, the percentage of women giving favorable assessments of their method of choice is lower for discontinuers than continuers, as one might expect. However, Norplant discontinuers were the most dissatisfied of the three groups: While the majority of former Depo-Provera and pill users would recommend "their" method to a friend, that was the case for only a minority of those who had had their implant removed. Nevertheless, both Norplant continuers and discontinuers, in similar proportions, valued the method's convenience and effectiveness; their reservations were focused almost entirely on menstrual and nonmenstrual side effects. At the same time, there was little difference between women who discontinued Norplant and those who discontinued Depo-Provera in their dislike of both menstrual and nonmenstrual side effects. Pill users, continuers and discontinuers alike, did not like taking the pill daily.

The Question of Coercion

Slightly over 15 percent of women who planned, considered, or actually proceeded to seek removal of the implant perceived pressure from a health care provider not to do so. For those women, the results were more and less satisfactory visits for removal than was the case for women who experienced no pressure. Despite this unfortunate statistic, such pressure, real or perceived, was insufficient to explain the much lower discontinuation rate associated with Norplant compared to the other two methods during this study.

Postdiscontinuation Experience

The study also addressed questions about what happens after discontinuation, since differences in the postdiscontinuation experience may contribute to the extended use-effectiveness of the methods that have been discontinued.

The patterns of behavior after discontinuation of each of the three methods studied proved, in fact, to be quite different. Almost no Norplant discontinuers switched to exposed non-use (not using a method but sexually active and not seeking pregnancy) and few switched to coitus-dependent methods (primarily condoms). In contrast, the proportions of Depo-Provera and pill users who switched to exposed non-use or use of a coitus-dependent method were much higher and roughly similar to each other. Among the reasons for this disparity may be that women who had chosen Norplant were more motivated to choose a highly effective method in the first place, or the provider on whom they had depended for implant removal may have counseled them to select another highly effective method.

When each group did opt for another effective method, Norplant users were most likely to turn to the pill and, next, Depo-Provera; no Norplant users sought sterilization. Depo-Provera users moved overwhelmingly to the pill, pill users moved overwhelmingly to Depo-Provera, and a small proportion of both groups sought sterilization. Only a small proportion of Depo-Provera users and pill users switched to Norplant. However, because of the small number of Norplant users who discontinued use and then switched to other contraceptive options, it is hard to develop a solid response to questions about the impact of switching on rates of unintended pregnancy.

Conclusions

Compared to users of Depo-Provera and the pill, Norplant users have a greater number of side effects and somewhat more severe side effects; they are also somewhat less satisfied. At the same time, Norplant users have the most effective contraceptive outcomes. They have the lowest discontinuation rate; are tied with Depo-Provera users in having the lowest use-failure (unintended pregnancy) rate; and, after discontinuing Norplant, are least likely to switch to exposed non-use and most likely to switch to an effective method. On balance, the results from this study indicate that Norplant is a most valuable tool to have in the armamentarium of contraceptives.

Presentation 10
THE ECONOMICS OF CONTRACEPTION
Felicia H. Stewart, M.D.
Henry J. Kaiser Family Foundation

Background

Beyond thinking about contraception from the standpoint of population growth or its role in reproductive health, there is an economic perspective that is useful for at least two reasons. One is that such a perspective offers a basis for greater public-sector investment in the provision of a full range of contraceptives for those without access to other avenues. The other is that it helps price current or prospective markets as a point of departure for greater industry involvement in contraceptive research and development. While it is surely true that the costs of high rates of unintended pregnancy are primarily human, social, and health costs rather than purely economic, the economic costs are substantial nonetheless and ought not be omitted from our thinking about contraception and contraceptives.

Methodology

The prime objective of this effort was to compare the costs of 15 categories of reversible and irreversible contraceptives. A computer model was developed to calculate a total cost for each. The model included the direct medical costs of using each method, as well as the medical costs and benefits associated with side effects, positive (e.g., protection against disease, based on incidence and relative risk) and negative (e.g., complications associated with method use, based on incidence and treatment costs).[*]

Then, assuming the typical use failure rate for each contraceptive method, the model calculated the costs of pregnancies occurring as a result of failure, based on the four possible unintended pregnancy outcomes—spontaneous abortion, ectopic pregnancy, induced abortion, or birth—each in the proportion expected nationally in the United States. These calculations did not include possible ancillary costs of unintended pregnancy such as welfare payments; Women, Infants, Children (WIC); and any subsequent disability. The assumption was made that no method switching occurred following unintended pregnancy. Costs were factored into the model only until a pregnancy outcome was resolved and were not incorporated following the birth of a child. All costs were derived from the Medicaid schedule of benefits for the state of California (Medi-Cal) and, for purposes of comparison, from a national private payer database (Medstat's Market Scan).

The model also incorporated assumptions about time horizons, since some contraceptive methods require a greater one-time (e.g., sterilization) or initial (e.g., implant) investment, which would bias a 1-year time frame considerably. Thus, periods of use of 1 through 5 years were calculated for all methods, together with their cumulative costs over 5 years, to locate the point at which investment in a given method would become cost-effective compared to use of no method or compared to the others.

Sexually transmitted diseases (STDs) were not included in the first iteration of this model, not because they were not deemed important but because in the general population of women aged 15 to 44, STD prevalence proved in sensitivity analysis not to make a meaningful difference in final cost-effectiveness estimates. However, in the next model iteration, refined to model costs for adolescents more appropriately, STDs and their associated treatment costs were included, and the assumption that some methods provide varying degrees of protection against STDs was factored into the cost-effectiveness equation. The model also used the higher failure rates that are reported for adolescents and omitted methods such as vasectomy, tubal ligation, and intrauterine devices that are less likely to be used by younger individuals.

---

[*] Lee PR, and FH Stewart. Editorial: Failing to prevent unintended pregnancy is costly. *American Journal of Public Health* 85(4):479–480, 1995. Trussell J, JA Leveque, JDD Koenig, et al. Documenting the economic value of contraception: A comparison of 15 methods. *American Journal of Public Health* 85(4):495–503, 1995b.

Findings

The cost-effectiveness conclusions resulting from both databases were very similar, with the Medicaid costs parallel, but somewhat lower overall than those derived from the private payer database. The results that follow are based on private payer costs.

The model was summarized in a series of bar graphs in which each method was represented by a bar consisting of estimated costs for: (1) method use (including medical services), the method itself, accessories (e.g., Norplant insertion kit), all based on estimated average number of uses annually; (2) adverse and beneficial side effects costs, including related clinical visits and treatment; and (3) unintended pregnancy costs, based on the typical failure rates for each method.

After adjusting for national averages for the four different pregnancy outcomes, individuals using the male condom for 5 years should factor in $2,400 to cover the costs of unintended pregnancy associated with use of that method; those using withdrawal, $3,300; and women using a diaphragm, $3,700, spermicide, $4,100, female condom, $4,900, and cervical cap, $5,700. The use of no method at all was determined to be a $14,700 investment for one woman over 5 years.

The reason for all this is that in the United States, pregnancy is not a thrifty undertaking; in a managed care setting, the costs of a birth for mother and baby are about $9,000. Thus, it is failure rates, their consequences in the form of unintended pregnancy, and the high price of pregnancy, that produce the primary costs for all contraceptive methods and determine their rank ordering in terms of cost-effectiveness.

A critical finding from these calculations is that tubal ligation, which competes with oral contraceptives as the most used method in the United States, fails to reach cost-effectiveness when compared to other methods by 5 years. This suggests the need to revise the prevailing notion that this method is somehow intrinsically preferable to other long-acting methods such as implants or injectables, especially given new data on higher failure rates for tubal ligation than previously anticipated, as well as the risk of ectopic pregnancy and method failure as long as 10 years postligation. Vasectomy, on the other hand, proves to be a highly cost-effective option.

Another interesting finding is how early the crossover into cost-effectiveness occurs for methods typically viewed as too expensive as a result of high initial cost. Norplant, for example, becomes more cost-effective than the injectable at 3 years of use. Of all long-acting reversible methods, the copper T IUD, appropriately prescribed, is the most thrifty.

Looking at the same cumulative cost issue for younger contraceptive users, specifically teenagers, the crossovers into cost-effectiveness for implants and injectables occur much earlier than might be expected, contrary to the perception that those methods are too expensive to be offered routinely to young people in clinics.

The teen model, which takes into account STD prevalence, treatment costs, and the risk reduction benefits of some methods, notably condoms and spermicides, also shows that STD costs contribute significantly to the overall cost of "no method" use.

The revised model also takes into account that for these age cohorts, a pregnancy prevented is, in most cases, delayed rather than averted. In the population as a whole, mis-timed births as opposed to unwanted births account for about 69 percent of the total number of unplanned pregnancies; for young people, that proportion is about 79 percent. The savings derived from delaying those births rather than avoiding them entirely, are the discounted costs over the 2-year delay of not spending the money now but, instead, spending it 2 years later. That makes the savings less: The cost over 5 years for a young person using no contraceptive method is about $8,000. The overall picture is, however, the same.

This sort of analysis—essentially a "savings" model—indicates that contraceptive methods with low failure rates are by far the most cost-effective, but that all methods of contraception are cost-effective compared to the costs of unintended pregnancy. In sensitivity analyses, this held true even for dual-method use: back-up methods such as emergency contraception or male condom use along with another "primary" method remain cost-effective. In other words, enough is saved by the additional reduction of unintended pregnancy or, for the youngest groups of contraceptors, disease prevention, to more than pay for the cost of providing both methods.

Conclusions

All this means that providing more comprehensive coverage, assuring that contraception is not something that individuals have difficulty getting, and not permitting initial investment cost to act as a barrier to use, are clearly cost-effective and thrifty approaches. However, in the United States, the manner in which health care systems are set up typically requires individuals to incur the method cost, while insurers incur the costs of pregnancy. This creates a situation where individuals are given incentives to select the least expensive contraceptive options which, paradoxically, are the least effective. This arrangement deserves careful scrutiny because of the tension, nonproductive in terms of health and well-being, between the potential for insurers to save money and the possibility that individuals will make less than optimal contraceptive choices.

Presentation 11
IMPLANT REMOVAL AND TRAINING
David Archer, M.D.
Jones Institute, Eastern Virginia Medical College

Background

Norplant's perhaps most significant limitation is that it requires a provider to insert and remove it. There are expenditures associated with these requirements and, while the costs of insertion may be clearly seen as part of the up-front costs of the method, the additional costs of removal are more problematic. That set of issues is addressed in the body of this workshop report.

Although both insertion and removal seem to be simple procedures, for virtually all providers there is a learning curve associated with putting the device in and taking it out. Done correctly, a proper insertion allows a provider to feel the capsules in a fan-like arrangement beneath the skin. These are the easiest removals. However, when the insertion has been poorly done, the capsules may be in uneven relationships with one another. This is generally not a problem while the implant remains *in situ* but it may well produce complications when a provider—often not the same provider who inserted it—attempts to remove it.

Removal Techniques

Three removal methods currently predominate: (1) standard, (2) pop-out, and (3) U techniques. For all methods, removal proceeds following injection with a local anesthetic near the base of the fan of capsules. Although numbness and blistering of the skin occur immediately, the anesthetic usually requires 5 to 7 minutes to take effect; a provider may rub the injection site to help disperse the anesthetic. There is usually some discomfort later when the anesthetic effect wanes, since fibrous connective tissue lining surrounds each implant capsule and is connected to subcutaneous tissue at the base of each capsule and at the distal end near the capsule shoulder.

Standard Technique

The earliest technique, used in Norplant introductory training in the United States, calls for an incision, at the base of the fan, large enough for a straight hemostat or forceps to enter. The provider breaks down some of the adhesions that have formed while the implant has been *in situ* so as to loosen each implant capsule and make it easily accessible. One hand then stabilizes the first capsule in the fan by pushing it down and, as the jaws of the hemostat open, the forefinger of the other hand is used to help guide the capsule and stabilize it into the hemostat.

APPENDIX A

The provider then pulls down and everts the hemostat, allowing the end of the capsule to be identified. Several steps follow: using a knife or scalpel to incise the capsule and, then, a hemostat or a gauze sponge to press the fibrous capsule to expose the Norplant capsule beneath the fibrous connective tissue and remove it. This is repeated for all six capsules.

This technique can be completed in 12 to 15 minutes but may take 30 minutes or more, owing to difficulty in feeling the Norplant capsules, capturing them, and bringing them to the incision site, particularly when they have been inserted poorly. Failure with the hemostat capture technique may cause the provider to attempt to grab the capsule, which is difficult to control and sometimes springs away. And, if the operator has used too much local anesthetic, palpation will be more difficult, causing further delay. A major challenge in removal training, using this technique or any other, is to make providers understand that when the removal is difficult and too much time passes—and 30 minutes is the limit—attempts at removal should halt because of almost inevitable swelling of tissue.

Pop-Out Technique

This technique requires more precision than the standard technique. After injecting anesthetic, the provider identifies the capsule by pressing down on it and "milking" it to the incision site so that the end of the capsule protrudes. This involves stabilizing the capsule with one hand (usually the left hand for a right-handed operator) and moving the skin over the top of the capsule, thus positioning it at the very small incision site. Once that is done and the fibrous capsule has been opened, the provider should be able to extrude each implanted capsule by seizing it with his or her fingers. Providers who use this technique say it can be done relatively expeditiously, but the precision required appears to take more time and skill than are typical for the average physician.

U Technique

This technique, named after its Indonesian inventor, Dr. Praptohardjo, removes the implanted capsules in a U-shaped fashion. The technique uses a modified vasectomy clamp that allows the provider to go around the entire Norplant device and capture it so that it becomes totally enclosed in the incision site. The incision is made between the third and fourth implant capsules so that an equal number of capsules are on either side and at the level of the middle of the capsules rather than at the base, because each capsule will need to be secured with the modified vasectomy clamp several millimeters from its tip. Again the capsules are identified and controlled with one hand, moving them into the jaws of the device. As the capsule is lifted, it "tents" and the device seizes around it, pulling it to the incision site and causing a tugging sensation that some individuals may experience as discomfort or pain. The provider then opens up the device higher on the fibrous capsule. Ultimately the provider will either flip out the short end, or grab it and bring it out in a J hook or a U shape, using a secondary hemostat for the actual removal. While the description of the procedure is complicated, the manual dexterity required is less than that needed for the standard technique, so that removal is likely to be easier and training is correspondingly simpler.

Removal Difficulties and Training

In the United States, because a fair number of devices had not been placed appropriately and capsules cannot always be located via palpation, providers have tried a variety of techniques for finding poorly inserted implants. These have included a compression mammogram to see the capsules better; however, although the devices are readily visible individually, it is hard to see them in relationship to one another because they move. Other providers have tried using triangulation or grids, but such two-dimensional approaches have not so far proved compatible with what is basically a three-dimensional task. Fluoroscopy has also been attempted, but proved too cumbersome.

Ultrasound, a technology readily available to many physicians and usable in an ambulatory outpatient facility, is suggested in the 1995 labeling (Prescribing Information), along with compression mammography. In a cross-sectional scan, the ultrasound wave is perpendicular or quasi-perpendicular to the plane of the set of implants; because the ultrasound wave is being reflected back to the scanning head, a shadow appears behind each capsule. However, the shortness of the wave length means that, to create a reasonable focal length, a distance must be established in the interface between the patient's skin and the scanner head. A small water-filled balloon or condom is used to accomplish this, but this is a fairly clumsy process in which the provider is scanning, trying to identify the capsules, and holding on to yet another elusive object at the same time. This technique and others mentioned may be helpful but they are far from ideal solutions.

Conclusions

The fundamental problem in difficult removals is poor insertion. When the device has been properly implanted, any trained provider should experience few problems in removing it using any of the techniques discussed. Providers must first accept that there is a learning curve for removal techniques and, second, that there are other associated skills that need to be acquired in training, including the counseling skills that will prepare patients appropriately for any discomfort during the removal process, particularly when it is expected to be difficult.

Presentation 12
IMPLANT REMOVAL AND TRAINING
Angela Davey
Hoechst Marion Roussel, Ltd., and
Lynne Gaffikin, Ph.D.
JHPIEGO Corporation

Background

The existence of a national health care system in the United Kingdom required an approach to the introduction of Norplant that was compatible with that system's philosophy and standard operating practices. Like all other pharmaceutical products provided through national health care, contraceptives are gratis to the patient. Pharmaceutical companies may disseminate product information only to physicians and are not allowed to talk or provide information to patients until the decision to prescribe a given product has been made by the provider, the "learned intermediary." Contraception and all reproductive health care are delivered at the primary care level, typically by a general practitioner long familiar with the patient's history. Only 10 percent of contraceptives are provided through family planning specialists, characteristically located in towns and cities and relatively few in number; the population of family planning specialists has fallen over the years owing to the belief that this service should be provided by general practitioners, a trend that is reversing somewhat as family planning services are increasingly seen as having something special to offer, especially for certain populations.

Three other contextual matters were relevant to the introduction of Norplant in the United Kingdom. One was the perception that progestin-only birth control methods, progestin-only pills (POP), and Depo-Provera were less desirable than other options and suitable only for small niche populations such as older women or women with special problems. This meant that physicians would need education about Norplant's distinguishing features so that it would not automatically be relegated to a minority role along with "other" progestin-only methods.

A second was, as in the United States, that aspect of medical culture that leads to the assumption that there is no need to learn what seem to be simple procedures and elementary messages. A similar assumption relates to the provider-client relationship and the content of counseling.

The final challenge to Norplant's success was money. Under national health care, general practitioners, who receive a fee for IUD insertions, get reimbursement for the insertion and removal of the contraceptive implant.

Methodology

The early information about Norplant that was available in the United Kingdom came from materials developed by Norplant's U.S. distributor, Wyeth-

Ayerst Research Laboratories. Because the United Kingdom had not been the site of clinical trials or pre-introductory studies and because no component of the implant was being produced there, there was no database of experience and locally generated information. In addition to a desire to have a better sense of the product overall, the conclusion after watching video material on insertion and removal was that successful introduction would depend on a general understanding of the product and its strengths and limitations, solid competency and confidence on the part of providers in insertion and removal, and appropriate client selection and counseling. To accomplish this, strong training efforts in all these areas would be essential, as would a locally generated body of "KAP" (Knowledge-Attitudes-Practices) data.

Norplant's distributor in the United Kingdom, Hoechst Marion Roussel, decided to build on the experience acquired through work in Indonesia by JHPIEGO, a training and technical assistance corporation largely funded by the U.S. Agency for International Development (USAID). The decision was made to utilize the expertise of U.S. and Indonesian trainers to train a small core of senior trainers on site in Indonesia, and then use those physicians to precipitate a "cascade" of training and one-on-one supervised clinical practice for a sequenced, targeted selection of providers in 35 training centers nationwide. A trainee checklist was developed to standardize the stages to competency in both insertions and removals and Hoechst Marion Roussel promised additional resources for support later to assist with any difficult removals. As noted previously, because pharmaceutical companies have no control at the point of delivery in the British health care system, there could be no insistence or guarantee that every clinician inserting Norplant had attended a workshop on insertion. In fact, however, the majority of general practitioners and family planning physicians did go through the training program and/or participated in workshops. Hoechst Marion Roussel also established a medical information support service, as well as routine follow-up visits to providers to discuss any problems or anticipated difficult removals.

A most important factor in the various processes of introduction and training were the very intimate links to pre-introductory market research. This research gathered data through interviews with providers and potential consumers which served to identify those populations for whom the method would be most appropriate and thereby determine what the market share would be. One important finding from that research was that, contrary to previous assumptions, Norplant was likely to be more attractive to a younger age bracket and less attractive to older women, originally forecast to be the primary user population.

The research also made it clear that method introduction would succeed or fail depending on the level of awareness among clinicians about the method, skills required to provide it optimally, use by women for whom it was appropriate, and the quality of counseling, especially the degree of clarity about the method's limitations as well as its value. Thus, the resources available for introducing Norplant were structured and focused to encompass all these factors. The information gathered further served as the basis for subsequent promotional campaigns and contributed to the development of high-quality support materials for physicians to distribute to their clients.

Findings

Another key element in the Norplant introduction strategy used in the United Kingdom was continuous postmarketing research, including two retrospective surveys, one with method users and one with clinicians, as well as a controlled clinical trial. A survey of women's attitudes toward Norplant concluded that counseling had been a crucial component in their experience with the method. Another survey was mailed to clinicians who had attended an insertion-and-removal workshop to determine continuation rates and reasons for removal. The survey found a very high continuation rate of 85 percent at 12 months, a rate equal to that found in the controlled clinical trial.

Conclusions

Overall, JHPIEGO considers the U.K. experience as a best-case scenario for method introduction, one that meticulously built on learning from what had been experienced elsewhere. Its most successful elements were the cascade training strategy, targeted selection of trainers at the start of the cascade, training of providers to the point of confidence and documented proficiency, heavy up-front emphasis on removals and their potential difficulties, supervised clinical practice, the clear linkages between pre-introductory market research and training, high-quality support materials, medical information support services, routine follow-up visits, continuous post-introduction research, and promotional campaigns.

All this excellence was not sufficient, however, to "immunize" the method against the sorts of contextual issues that have affected its use in other settings. The most vexing local matter was compensation to physicians for IUD insertion but not for Norplant, which became such a prominent concern for the practitioner unions that, in 1995, the General Medical Services Committee recommended that doctors stop inserting and removing Norplant until the question was sorted out. The British media picked up on the subject and method adoptions started to fall. The extensive negative coverage of litigation in the U.S. media is also thought to have contributed to an increase in implant removals.

Presentation 13
IMPLANT REMOVAL AND TRAINING
Paul Blumenthal, M.D.
Johns Hopkins University Bayview Medical Center

Background

With the advent of Norplant in the United States, the Bayview Medical Center in Baltimore, Maryland, opted to adopt a structured training program where practitioners would acquire competency in the method before advancing to training in a clinical setting. The decision to do this derived from knowledge of difficulties experienced in other countries, from the desire to profit from the experience of the JHPIEGO Corporation's training program in Indonesia and later in the United Kingdom, and from understandings about the way clinical procedures are taught in the United States. Before putting Norplant on the U.S. market, its distributor, Wyeth-Ayerst, provided support for a national hands-on training program in Norplant insertion for physicians, nurse practitioners, and physicians' assistants, using master trainers in 37 hospital- and clinic-based locations.

As unprecedented as it was for a pharmaceutical company to sponsor such an endeavor, the effort was affected by factors that had more to do with predominant medical culture and training traditions in the United States than anything else. First, for the most part, it had to be left to individual practitioners to present themselves for training since there was no way of requiring that they do so. Second was the indeterminate number of physicians who believe they already command enough basic skills to cope with new technical requirements that seem elementary, leaving them not motivated to find time in inevitably demanding schedules for training. Third, medical training, undergraduate or postgraduate, is often provided in circumstances where competency need not be demonstrated, documented, or required before use, an acute limitation when students are unenthusiastic about needing to be in the classroom in the first place.

Fourth, the prevailing pattern is that individual practitioners, once exposed to a surgical technique, adapt it as they will, which produces an enormous amount of variability in practice. Finally, in very specific terms, at the time of its U.S. introduction the experience with Norplant, especially removals, was not as deep or extensive in the United States as it was elsewhere, notably Indonesia. Nor was there an effort to replicate the strategy used in the United Kingdom, which had chosen to prepare its master trainers on site in Indonesia, because of the experience acquired in the preintroductory period in that country.

Methodology

Medical education in the United States traditionally emphasizes the transmission of information; students are evaluated according to the amount of information absorbed. Most training in clinical procedure occurs via exposure to a technique, followed by freedom to adapt it to suit practitioner preference; heterogeneity of practice is inevitable.

In contrast, the Baltimore training program, adapted from that developed by the JHPIEGO Corporation, emphasized transmission of skills and evaluation of performance. It also emphasized standardization: of those skills, the way they would be transmitted, and the eventual performance of trainees. The Baltimore group adapted a set of essential steps, to achieve technical consensus among their faculty on how insertion and removal would be performed and to standardize these agreed upon techniques so that training and skills assessment would be consistent throughout.

The one requirement of practitioners recruited to the program was a clear willingness to learn procedures and to practice them repeatedly. Those who intended to become trainers were required in addition to complete a course on skill acquisition and to demonstrate proficiency before being permitted to train others. Levels of skill acquisition and proficiency were defined and a checklist developed to guide trainees and those responsible for evaluating their performance. Parameters for handling procedurally difficult removals were set and accounted for during training.

One useful mechanism was development of the "VAP"—Visibility, Arrangement, Palpability—score for standardizing the assessment of the degree of difficulty of a prospective implant removal and anticipating the amount of time needed for the eventual procedure. A scale of 1 to 3 was established, with 1 indicating that all capsules or rods are visible, arrangement occurs in a fan-shaped distribution, and all implants are easily palpable with minimal pressure. Scores of 2 and 3 indicate graded complications within each of these characteristics.

Findings

The predominant client population in Baltimore for Norplant is young and many are teenagers. The pattern of requests for removal was a peak at 6 months, when most users have not yet experienced the settling down of menstrual irregularities that occurs in most women between 6 to 9 months. "Problem visits" to clinics generally cease after 6 months, because those who remain are generally satisfied or willing to tolerate side effects and those who are not have elected to have the implant removed. Experience with these removals proved that the VAP score did correlate with duration of procedure and was considered a good tool for predicting the time required for implant removal; it also proved useful in predicting difficult removals. The standardized procedure that had been developed for removal was found to require, on average, 15 minutes.

There were two provider populations at the center: physicians and physicians' assistants. One limited assessment found that mean removal time was longer for a physician who had not attended any formal training course and was essentially self-taught, than it was for a physician's assistant who took the course.

The shorter removal time was also found to have a positive effect on patient attitudes, thought to be vulnerable to the influence of ongoing media coverage of difficult removal experiences. Patient perceptions about the level of removal difficulty also coincided more closely with the perceptions of physicians' assistants than they did with those of physicians. Finally, the speed of the removal procedure correlated strikingly with the extent to which users, even though they had had the implant removed, would still recommend the method to a friend; the perception of the very large majority of these women was that their removal experience was much easier than they had anticipated.

Conclusions

Another contributor to method success and improved removal experiences will be the removal technique itself. The "U" method of removal was developed and evaluated in Indonesia as a possible alternative method. Mean removal times were calculated for the standard and the U techniques in a total of 250 removals, and the number of removals required for initial and sustained competency was evaluated. Initial competency was defined as fulfilling all the required steps at least once and was assessed to determine whether a practitioner fell back to "incompetency" before his or her competency could be said to be sustained. The result was that sustained competency could be achieved an average of two patients sooner using the U technique; removal times with that technique were also significantly lower and with a smaller percentage of removal problems. Since removal time seems to be inextricably linked to overall patient perception of the method, any removal technology that could expedite removal and therefore improve client perceptions is very desirable.

The Baltimore training and clinical experience demonstrated that client attitudes toward Norplant and, ultimately, use of the method in general, can be modified by provision of safe and expedient removal. For the method to be a popular contraceptive option for women, removals need to be provided by competent, well-trained personnel with experience involving a variety of levels of difficulty.

Another critical variable would be standardization of implant insertion and removal procedures. At a recent symposium sponsored by Wyeth-Ayerst, participants discussed the possibility of establishing a certification requirement for the insertion and removal of Norplant but concluded that such a propostion was unlikely to gain favor. However, some degree of standardizing the procedures was considered both worthwhile and feasible.

APPENDIX A

Presentation 14
INTRODUCTION OF NORPLANT INTO INDONESIA
Ruth Simmons, Ph.D.
University of Michigan
School of Public Health

Background

In 1989, when Norplant moved from the research stage into full-scale introduction in Indonesia, many difficulties ensued. To prepare for introduction, the Population Council that same year performed a small study in three provinces of Indonesia focusing on quality of service delivery, in particular on three critical factors: (1) choice, that is, whether women accepting Norplant were given a choice among a range of methods and could make their eventual choice freely; (2) whether removal on demand was available; and (3) the extent to which the Indonesia program was capable of ensuring 5-year removal tracking.

Findings

Choice

Evaluation of the Indonesian program found that choice was not consistently realized. Across the entire program, women's access to information was limited, both with respect to the implant technology itself and alternative method options. Beyond the general tendencies of providers to be authoritative in their guidance and brief with their time, the belief prevailed that women did not need much information, a belief reinforced by a national policy of emphasizing long-acting methods and by the fact that sterilization is negatively sanctioned for religious reasons. Not only was that policy well known but field staff and providers were rewarded for the number of women they recruited to all those methods, including Norplant.

These factors were further reinforced by the community-based campaign style of the method's introduction. Much effort went into mobilizing communities to accept the premise that this was the method that women should adopt, and community buildings and schools became the sites of mass efforts to provide insertions, typically under considerable time pressure.

Removal on Demand

The second critical element identified in the Population Council study was removal on demand. Removal on demand had been assured during field trials when, quite rightly, program managers welcomed the need for training in removal techniques. However, as the method went to full-scale introduction through the national program, women were often given the message that they were making a 5-year commitment and women who later sought to have the implant removed earlier than that were likely to encounter provider reluctance and resistance.

Tracking Capacity

Even though program managers recognized that not enough providers had been appropriately trained in removal skills, the assumption was that the program basically had 5 years in which to catch up in this regard. When the 5 years were up, concerns about the national program's capacity for tracking adopters proved justified. That capacity was at best uneven and particularly challenged in dense urban areas. Furthermore, the national program could not count on women showing up for removal of their own accord at the end of Norplant's 5-year period of approved efficacy, since it was not at all clear that most women had received enough information at the time of insertion to appreciate the importance of removal 5 years later.

In addition, the study identified several problems related to the technical quality of care. The reasons were many: the sheer volume of activity, the pressures of time, the fact that many providers were inadequately prepared in insertion and removal techniques, equipment and supplies were inadequate, and maintenance of an aseptic environment was not a priority.

Program evaluation discovered serious problems that emerged when Norplant went to scale. The difficulties were philosophical and strategic, perhaps the natural result of pushing women toward a particular method rather than helping them make choices among methods. The difficulties were also administrative and technical. Launching a brand new, complex contraceptive method for use by large numbers of women in a short period of time would compromise the quality of care and provider-client interaction in most delivery systems, even more so given the cultural constraints and limited resources in the Indonesian program.

Conclusions

The Indonesian experience, together with lessons from IUD introduction in India in the early years of the method, as well as more recent lessons from Cyclofem introduction in Indonesia, prompted the World Health Organization (WHO) to develop a new program designed to avoid repetition of errors. The foundation of the approach is a broad assessment of key factors before a decision is made to introduce a method: this has already affected the ways in which some countries are making decisions about introducing new methods and overall method mix. Vietnam, for instance, reversed itself on a decision to introduce Norplant, and instead decided to focus more systematically on improving quality of care through the introduction of injectables and to hold off on Norplant introduction until quality of care can be better assured. It is reasonable to expect that, as a general matter, optimal system preparation should head off many of the problems that seem to attend the introduction of contraceptive methods, whatever they are.

Presentation 15
LOOKING TO THE FUTURE
A FEDERAL STANDARDS DEFENSE:
WHAT DIFFERENCE MIGHT IT MAKE?[1]
Michael D. Green, J.D.
College of Law, University of Iowa

Background

In considering whether a federal standards defense might have made a difference in the case of Norplant, two areas are especially germane: (1) efforts already made to address product liability at both the state and federal levels, and (2) the role and capacity of the Food and Drug Administration (FDA).

A number of states have enacted some form of regulatory approval defense that is specific to pharmaceuticals. Of those, Michigan law is the most protective, providing that there is no liability for any drug that has been approved by the FDA, as long as no fraud or bribery has been involved in obtaining premarketing approval from that agency.[2]

At the federal level, a regulatory approval defense was included in the House version of the Common Sense Products Liability and Legal Reform Act of 1995 but was removed in conference as part of a compromise strategy for avoiding a presidential veto; the veto occurred and the attempt at an override failed.[3] The experience with this piece of legislation serves to highlight a major consideration, that is, the extent to which the entire topic of products liability is politicized and the breadth of legal, regulatory, industrial, and consumer interests at play in this particular arena.

Discussion

The Role of the FDA

Much of the strength of a regulatory approval defense rests on the processes of oversight by the FDA that are intended to assure compliance by manufacturers with the agency's regulations, both in the premarketing and postmarketing periods. During the premarketing phases, manufacturers must comply with FDA regulations for adequate and well-controlled studies, accurate reporting of results, and truthful responses to inquiries from the agency associated with New Drug Application (NDA) review. The FDA, in turn, depends for its decisions about product approvals on extensive preclinical and clinical trials that are carried out either by the manufacturer or a contract research organization hired by the manufacturer to assure product safety and efficacy. Oversight of data collection in clinical settings may be carried out by monitors hired by the manufacturer to assure the quality and integrity of the data and the process of its collection. The data required are typically complex and amounts may be massive. For example, the New Drug Application (NDA) for Norplant consisted of 53 volumes of data and analysis.

In addition, there are some tensions among the various incentives for industry compliance with FDA requirements that have to do with the costs of testing, in time and money; pressures for approval so as to get a product to market, especially first to market; and the goal that all product risks be fully identified.

FDA's capabilities for fulfilling its responsibilities are substantial and constitute the strongest case for a regulatory standards defense. The agency customarily, and increasingly, does an accurate and reliable job during this period, surpassing what can be accomplished on a regular basis through the present tort system because of the technical expertise resident on the agency's staff, as well as available through its advisory committees. Furthermore, the flexibile FDA decision-making processes are quite different from the adversarial model of the tort system, as are its processes for assessing relative risks and benefits.

The postmarketing period is more problematic and raises issues that are critical for conceptualizing a government standards defense.[4] Many adverse reactions simply cannot be identified within the time frames and samples customary for premarketing trials and will emerge only after market introduction as the experienced population increases in size and heterogeneity. A 1990 General Accounting Office study found that of the 198 drugs approved between 1976 and 1985 for which data were available, 102 (51.5 percent) had serious postapproval risks, as evidenced by labeling changes on 96 drugs and removal from the market of 6 drugs. The large majority of the drugs were deemed by the FDA to have benefits outweighing their risks, so that resulting label changes either limited the intended target population for the drug or required addition of major precautionary warnings regarding its use.[5] When clinical trials have been well designed and executed and the resulting data have been fully and openly reported to the FDA, later discoveries of adverse reactions are "no one's fault." However, reasonable prospects for such discoveries mean that well-designed, well-executed postmarketing surveillance becomes crucial. In this connection, it is also important for manufacturers to gather and report on adverse events so that risk can be identified and communicated and necessary modifications to labeling can be effected expeditiously. The role of labeling in protecting companies from liability is substantial.

The Potential Role of a Federal Standards Defense

There is little disagreement about these realities but there is a range of opinions about their implications for developing the sort of defense proposed in the 1990 and 1996 IOM committee reports,[6] and pros and cons abound. For example, one interpretation is that a government standards defense might dilute manufacturer interest in reporting adverse events in the postmarketing period because such a defense would have been predicated on data from the premarketing period. An alternative view is that incorporating a postmarketing surveillance requirement into the defense would be an appropriate hedge against such an eventuality and that, in any case, pharmaceutical companies already tend to see such surveillance as prudent and desirable. Furthermore, the FDA already requires reports of adverse events as a matter of course. Looking more broadly, another thought is that a government standards defense might motivate attorneys to probe more deeply into the thoroughness and integrity of company compliance with FDA requirements, rather than to take FDA approval at face value. The effect might be to increase incentives to push such determinations into the courtroom more frequently, an eventuality some might find unappealing.

The question was posed as to whether some kind of federal standards defense might have constituted a deterrent to the kind of litigation seen in connection with Norplant. The claims related to Norplant have been for relatively modest injuries, for example, difficulties related to removal, alleged norgestrel-related effects, and silastic-related claims. Thus, something like Michigan's product liability legislation might have had a substantial deterrent effect. Even though such provisions might not provide complete immunity from suit, claims for modest injuries would probably be filtered out, although claims for more serious injuries, such as birth defects, would still be likely to generate suits. This interpretation is, of course, hypothetical, suggesting that an empirical study of state-level product liability laws and their effects would be useful, perhaps essential, if the concept of a federal standards defense is to be addressed further.

Another related, bottom-line and, in effect, hypothetical question is whether such legislation would, in fact, encourage companies to re-enter or remain in the contraceptives market. The prevalent wisdom in the field continues to be that the threats of litigation and damaged corporate image are what have chilled industrial interest in contraceptive research and development. However, a number of studies have concluded that the incidence of punitive damage awards against pharmaceutical companies that have become final after all appeal are much lower than is generally perceived.[7] Still, the sheer perception of the risk of such damages, with their unpredictably high costs, both in dollars and goodwill lost, persists as a significant factor in pharmaceutical R&D decision-making nevertheless and, although this might be seen as overreaction to what have been found by some analysts to be relatively rare events, the perception in itself appears to be powerful and durable. Whether a workable government standards defense could remove that chill yet maintain incentives for compliance with FDA standards, especially for post-approval risks, and permit reasonable compensation in those instances when a manufacturer's noncompliance creates real risks, is difficult to know. The proof would necessarily have to be in the testing, that is, the actual adoption of such a reform. With regard to the general hypothetical question, as well as the particulars of such a reform, the issues are more complicated than many observers and commentators may have appreciated.

Finally, there is the issue of the scope of the defense in question and which approach might be most effectively applied to contraceptives, or at least subsume them. There are several options for consideration: a defense for all consumer products that must meet government standards; a defense limited to FDA-approved pharmaceuticals; or a narrow defense targeted to a specific product group for which there is a widely and urgently perceived need that is likely to rally constituency for protective legislation.

Two examples of the last category are the General Aviation Revitalization Act of 1994 and the National Children's Vaccine Act of 1986 and the associated National Vaccine Injury Compensation Program (VICP) implemented in 1988. The Revitalization Act was enacted to reduce the liability faced by aviation manufacturers, perceived as having substantially reduced R&D investment, with consequent negative effects on R&D advances, product quality, export potential, and employment. The VICP is a federal no-fault system designed to provide compensation to those injured by childhood vaccines, whether administered in the private or public sector. It came into being because of a decrease in the number of vaccine-producers owing to liability claims concerning adverse events, and because of apprehension about the effects of that diminution on supplies of existing vaccines and on new vaccine R&D. The program is generally believed to have had salutary effects in these regards. The question of the scope of a statutory corrective that would encompass contraceptives remains unresolved.

ENDNOTES

1. Two Institute of Medicine committees studying contraceptive research and development in 1990 and 1996 recommended that the U.S. Congress enact a federal product liability statute that would make FDA approval of contraceptive drugs and devices available to contraceptive manufacturers as a defense to punitive damages, assuming proper compliance with FDA regulatory requirements. Both committees contended that for controversial products that contribute importantly to the public health yet produce only modest profit margins, limits on liability could act as an incentive for research and development or at least could reduce the amount of disincentive. The 1990 committee argued that pharmaceuticals and medical devices are unique among products in the United States in the degree to which quality is regulated before they are released in the market, so that the need for liability as a quality control mechanism is greatly reduced (National Research Council and Institute of Medicine. *Developing New Contraceptives: Obstacles and Opportunities*. L Mastroianni Jr, PJ Donaldson, TT Kane, eds. Washington, DC: National Academy Press, 1990; Institute of Medicine. *Contraceptive Research and Development: Looking to the Future*. PF Harrison, and A Rosenfield, eds. Washington, DC: National Academy Press, 1996).

As conceptualized by that committee, with such a statute—variously referred to as a federal, government, or regulatory standards defense; regulatory approval or compliance defense; or simply as an "FDA defense"—companies would not be held liable for punitive damages in a lawsuit under the following assumptions: if the drug or medical device involved had received approval from the FDA and if that company had fully complied with all of the agency's requirements for premarketing testing and postmarketing surveillance. The defense would not, however, bar plaintiffs from obtaining compensatory damages. Nor

APPENDIX A

would it be available to a manufacturer found to have withheld from the FDA either information gathered for purposes of premarketing approval, or information developed after approval for review so as to determine whether the product in question, its marketing, or its labeling should be modified. Some have expressed the view that *any* violation of the comprehensive regulatory scheme overseen by the FDA that might be causally related to pharmaceutical injury would fall outside the scope of an FDA compliance defense. In other words, a consumer injured by a pharmaceutical or medical device would be free to recover compensatory and punitive damages if the injury would not have occurred if the manufacturer had complied fully with all FDA regulations.

2. Arizona, Colorado, New Jersey, Ohio, Oregon, and Utah have passed legislation that allows the manufacturer of an FDA-approved product to assert a government standards defense in response to claims for punitive damages. In addition, Illinois and North Dakota have adopted a defense to punitive or exemplary damages for products that have been approved by a state or federal regulatory agency with authority to approve the product in question (Institute of Medicine, op. cit., 1996).

3. The regulatory approval defense included in the House version (H.R. 956) of the 1995 bill barred punitive damages in cases where a medical device or drug had won premarketing approval from the FDA. H.R. 956 also capped punitive damages, at either $250,000 or at three times any economic losses, and was written to be applicable to any civil litigation, not just product disputes. The Senate version (S. 565) did not include a regulatory approval defense; also capped punitive damages at $250,000 or three times economic losses, but defined the latter as the greater of lost wages or medical expenses; and applied only to product liability cases (Institute of Medicine, op. cit., 1996). However, the compromise legislation that emerged from conference was vetoed and failed to muster enough votes to override.

4. The 1990 IOM committee, in recommending enactment of a federal product liability statute, spoke frankly on the inadequacy of existing postmarketing surveillance systems for contraceptive products and on the ethical, practical, and economic obstacles to successful postmarketing surveillance. That committee recommended establishment of a comprehensive postmarketing surveillance system to provide systematic and timely feedback about positive and negative health effects of contraceptive products. In addition, both the 1990 and 1996 committees noted that because a regulatory standards defense would necessarily interact with postmarketing surveillance efforts, any recommendation for such a statute would be more compelling were formal postmarketing surveillance studies to be an integral and general requirement.

5. U.S. General Accounting Office. *FDA Drug Review: Postapproval Risks 1976–1985 (Report of the Chairman, Subcommittee on Human Resources and Intergovernmental Relations, Committee on Government Operations, House of Representatives)*. Washington, D.C.: General Accounting Office, Program Evaluation and Methodology Division, 1990.

6. Institute of Medicine, *op. cit.,* 1990 and 1996.

7. MD Green. Statutory compliance and tort liability: Examining the strongest case. *University of Michigan Journal of Law Reform* 30(2&3), Winter–Spring, 1997). See also: S Daniels, and J Martin. Myth and reality in punitive damages. 75 *Minnesota Law Review* 1:28–43, 1990; MJ Saks. Do we really know anything about the behavior of the tort litigation system—And why not? 140 *University of Pennsylvania Law Review* 1147:1254–1262, 1992; S Garber. *Product Liability and the Economics of Pharmaceuticals and Medical Devices*. Santa Monica, CA: The Rand Corporation, 1993.

B

Norplant: Historical Background

THE TECHNOLOGY

The Norplant® implant system is a long-acting, reversible contraceptive consisting of six slim, small, flexible Silastic®[1] capsules, each containing 36 mg. of the hormone levonorgestrel. These are inserted in a fan-like pattern just under the skin of a woman's upper arm in an office-based surgical procedure under local anesthesia, and removed in similar fashion. The capsules slowly and steadily diffuse the levonorgestrel, which is a potent synthetic progestin with some androgenic activity and which prevents pregnancy through several modes of action: altering the cervical mucus to prevent penetration by sperm; inhibiting ovulation; changing the corpus luteum function; and suppressing the endometrium.[2] Duration of documented efficacy is 5 years, at which point the overall effectiveness of the implant starts to decline slowly and removal is necessary. The early goals of implant technology were to identify systems that would avoid first passage through the liver (as is the case with oral contraceptives [OCs]) and to develop a continuous release system that would avoid daily surges of hormone.

Norplant was the first implantable contraceptive introduced onto the world market, but other progestin only implant systems have been developed more or less in parallel, differing in the biomaterial used for the delivery system, steroid contents, number of implanted rods or capsules, primary mode of action, and duration of efficacy. None of these implant systems is yet on the market in any country.[3] Only one—the LNG ROD, a two-rod levonorgestrel implant system, informally referred to as "Norplant-2"—has been approved by the Food and Drug Administration (FDA). Decisions about its availability depend on assessments of market conditions by Wyeth-Ayerst and Leiras Oy, the U.S. and European companies with the rights to distribute it.[4] The two-rod implant provides drug

---

The material in this appendix was not presented at the workshop. It was prepared by staff as background for the reader and has been reviewed for accuracy.

release and clinical performance identical to that of the six-rod presentation but has a 3-year term of efficacy. The two-rod system was actually to have been the first implant launched on the U.S. market but, while trials were under way, the supplier ceased manufacture of the elastomer used in the core of the Norplant-2 implant and a change of plans was required.[5]

Definitions of advantages and disadvantages of any contraceptive method are partly subjective, dependent as they are on individual physiology and context but, in general, the inherent advantages and disadvantages of progestin implants as a contraceptive category are as follows:

- *Advantages:* extremely high efficacy; estrogen-free protection; low and stable blood level maintenance; freedom from need for daily compliance; rapid return to previous fertility; no interference with coitus; no manipulation of genital area; easy palpation; and long duration of action.
- *Disadvantages:* requirement for minor surgical procedures for insertion and removal; lack of dosage titration; bleeding irregularities (prolonged bleeding, spotting, or amenorrhea); mood alterations (e.g., depression); visibility of implant; possible local scar formation; and, as with all methods other than condoms, no protection from sexually transmitted infection.

HISTORY

The intersectoral research and development process that brought Norplant onto the world market began in the mid-1960s, with articulation by the Population Council of the general concept and objectives of implant technologies. In December 1990, after 25 years of development, FDA approval was granted. The process involved three major players and total costs of over $110 million:

- *Population Council:* research, $23.5 million; introduction into developing countries, $16 million
- *Leiras Oy:* development of manufacturing procedures, an estimated $23 million
- *Wyeth-Ayerst:* introduction into private sector, an estimated $50 million.[6]

Preparation for regulatory approval and eventual introduction of Norplant began in the early 1980s. The Population Council devised its introduction strategy in 1982 and began clinical trials and, later, preintroduction studies, in countries ranging from minimally to highly industrialized. It also licensed Norplant to Leiras Oy, a pharmaceutical company in Finland, the first country to approve the method. By 1988, over 55,000 women had had experience with Norplant through trials and studies in 41 countries (see Table B-1). These women were followed during the subsequent decade through over 70 user-acceptability studies conducted by the Council and other agencies in 20 countries,[7] which investigated method use and continuation, quality of care and counseling services, provider training, provider-client communication, adopter follow-up, access to the product and its removal, and overall satisfaction.

APPENDIX B

TABLE B-1 Trials Undertaken in Development of Norplant

Clinical Trials in 15 Countries:

1975–1979	Phase III multinational trials in Brazil, Chile, Denmark, Dominican Republic, Finland, Jamaica (PC/ICCR)
1980–1982	Trials begin in Colombia, Ecuador, Egypt, India, Indonesia, Thailand (PC)
1982	Phase II/III studies begin in the United States
	Another multinational Phase III clinical trial begins in Chile, Dominican Republic, Finland, Sweden, and the United States (PC/ICCR)
1990–1995	Phase III clinical trials of soft tubing Norplant capsules and reformulated Norplant with two rods in Chile, Dominican Republic, Egypt, Finland, Singapore, Thailand, United States

Preintroduction Studies in 30 Countries (start dates):

1984	Bangladesh, Brazil, Chile, China, Dominican Republic, Haiti, Kenya, Nepal, Nigeria
1985	Philippines, Singapore, Sri Lanka, Zambia
1988	Colombia, El Salvador, Ghana, Malaysia, Mexico, Pakistan, Peru, Senegal, South Korea, Tunisia, Venezuela, Zambia
1989	Bahamas, Rwanda, Zaire
1990	Bolivia, Madagascar

Private Sector Training in 7 Countries (Leiras Oy):

1988	Belgium, Bulgaria, former Soviet Union, France, Israel, West Germany, Taiwan

Postmarketing Surveillance in 8 Countries (WHO/HRP, PC, FHI):

1988–present	Bangladesh, Chile, China, Colombia, Egypt, Indonesia, Sri Lanka, Thailand

Training Curriculum Testing:
Nigeria, Rwanda, Kenya

International Training Centers:
Dominican Republic, Egypt, Indonesia

Regional Training Center:
Kenya

>70 Acceptability Studies in 20 Countries (FHI, PC, PATH, clinics, health ministries):

1987–present	Bangladesh, Brazil, China, Colombia, Dominican Republic, Ecuador, Egypt, Haiti, Indonesia, Kenya, Mexico, Nepal, Nigeria, Peru, Philippines, Rwanda, Sri Lanka, Thailand, United States, Zambia

NOTE: FHI = Family Health International; ICCR = International Committee for Contraception Research; PATH = Program for Appropriate Technologies in Health; PC = Population Council.

According to a World Bank consultation in 1995, the introduction of Norplant would be the first time a new contraceptive would be made available in developing countries through a systematic effort that explicitly set out to address the needs of both users and providers. The new approach was meant, first, to build on the lessons learned from introduction of the intrauterine device (IUD) in one large country site where lack of appropriate provider training and counseling about side effects had contributed to declining interest and discontinuation of use; second, to incorporate greater awareness of user perspectives toward voluntary and informed choice; and third, to ensure that family planning programs would be able to deliver services properly. The introduction strategy focused on: 1) developing local experience with the method through preintroduction trials aimed at offering firsthand experience to clinicians; 2) using trial sites as bases for developing in-country networks of training centers for future method expansion; 3) use of the data gathered to improve counseling materials and strategies; and 4) more comprehensive assessment of user needs and concerns, as well as service delivery requirements for expanding introduction. At the Twelfth World Congress of the Federation for International Gynecology and Obstetrics (FIGO), the then-director of the WHO/HRP observed that "probably no other contraceptive on the market [had] been developed by research done on such a large scale and reported step-by-step to the scientific community."

By the end of 1992, 24 countries had granted regulatory approval to Norplant; by mid-1995, that number had risen to 53; and by April 1997 it was 58,[8] with over 70 countries worldwide having had some experience with the method. Numbers of implants sold rose accordingly. As of the end of 1996, over 5 million units had been distributed, about 3.6 million of those in Indonesia and close to 1 million in the United States.

In the United States, where Wyeth-Ayerst had provided funding support for the training of some 27,000 clinicians in the techniques of implant insertion, removal, and appropriate counseling, insertions moved briskly after introduction of the method in February 1991. In Norplant's first full year on the U.S. market, sales reached $141 million, insertions were running at about 800 per day and, by the beginning of 1993, 1 million U.S. women had become Norplant users.[9]

In March 1994, negative coverage in the English- and Spanish-language U.S. media regarding women's problems with Norplant and initiation of lawsuits against Wyeth-Ayerst began to affect the market. The impetus for litigation came from a suit filed in Chicago in March 1994 on behalf of women who had experienced difficult implant removals. This was followed by negative media coverage, legal actions by attorneys for breast implant plaintiffs who filed similar complaints, and later filings by other plaintiffs' lawyers. Allegations of injury fell roughly into three categories:

• Removal difficulties, including capsule displacement, lengthy removals, or improper insertion
• Possible levonorgestrel-related effects, including acne, headache, depression, fatigue, mood swings, weight gain, weight loss, excessive bleeding,

ovarian cysts, increased intracranial hypertension, premature birth, birth defects, and other hormonal-related injuries

• Silastic-related claims, including autoimmune problems and other injuries alleged to be related to the silicone elastomer tubing containing the levonorgestrel.

In late summer 1995, the FDA affirmed support for Norplant in written testimony before the U.S. House of Representatives Committee on Government Reform and Oversight, Subcommittee on Human Resources and Intergovernmental Relations[10] but by 1996, annual U.S. sales of Norplant had dropped to $3.7 million and insertions had decreased by 90 percent.[11]

As of August 1997, 50,000 U.S. women nationwide were reported to have sued Wyeth-Ayerst, alleging that it failed to adequately warn users of side effects ranging from headaches and weight gain to ovarian cysts and depression. In addition, 2,800 lawsuits involving about 30,000 women were pending in a Beaumont, Texas, federal court but, as of that date no motion for consolidation of suits as class actions had been granted and no individual award had been made. On August 8, the Texas Supreme Court issued an order indefinitely delaying the trial set for August 11 that was to hear the suits brought by eight Texas women against Wyeth-Ayerst, so that the court could consider a motion by Wyeth attorneys to have several plaintiffs' attorneys disqualified for alleged misconduct.[12] While the principal defendant has been American Home Products and/or its subsidiary, Wyeth-Ayerst Laboratories, there have been suits against individual physicians and health care providers (including Planned Parenthood) involved in insertion or removal of the implant and/or treatment; manufacturer Leiras Oy or its parent company, Huhtamaki Oy;[13] Dow Corning or other Dow entities supplying the silastic tubing; Schering AG, the European supplier of bulk levonorgestrel; and the Population Council.

ENDNOTES

1. Dimethylsiloxane/methylvinylsiloxane copolymer. The capsules are sealed with silastic (polydimethylsiloxane) adhesive.

2. MF McCann, and LS Potter. Progestin-only oral contraception. A comprehensive review. *Contraception* 50(Suppl 1):9–S195, 1994.

3. The "second-generation" progestin-only implant systems include:

• Two-rod levonorgestrel implant system, tested since 1981, developed by the Population Council, and manufactured by Leiras Oy of Finland, the system was approved by the FDA on 15 August 1996 as safe and effective for 3 years of contraceptive use.

• Nestorone™, a single-rod implant with a core that is half silastic, half hormone, effective for 2 years, currently in clinical trials.

• Implanon, a single implant made of ethylene vinylacetate, containing 3-keto desogestrel, effective for 3 years, undergoing large-scale testing.

- Uniplant, a single silastic implant containing nonegestrol acetate, effective for 1 year, manufactured in Brazil and distributed by South-to-South but not yet registered in any country.

Similarly administered, each of these steroids affects target organs somewhat differently. For example, Norplant produces thickening of the cervical mucus that impedes sperm penetration, the mode of action that seems to contribute most to its high efficacy; this effect is much weaker with Nestorone, whose primary effect appears to be ovulation prevention (World Bank/Population Council/World Health Organization Special Program on Research, Development, and Research Training in Human Reproduction. *International Consultation on Contraceptive Implants* [unpublished paper]. Washington, D.C.: World Bank, 19 July 1995).

4. Wyeth-Ayerst is reported to be engaged in research and development related to an insertion device and is monitoring the U.S. contraceptive market to determine when a product launch might be feasible (A Ashby. Wyeth-Ayerst Laboratories Press Release: Statement on the FDA Approval of the Two-Rod Levonorgestrel Implant. Philadelphia, 15 August 1996). Leiras Oy, purchased by Schering AG in 1996, is taking time to develop a marketing strategy before making the product available (Program on Appropriate Technology for Health [PATH]. U.S. approves implant, availability unclear. *Outlook* 15[1]:7–8, June 1997). There are no indications from either company as to when, or whether, either is prepared to make the product available.

5. Sivin I, O Viegas, I Campodonico, et al. Clinical performance of a new two-rod levonorgestrel contraceptive implant: A three-year randomized study with Norplant[R] implants as controls. *Contraception* 55:73–80, February 1997.

6. Bardin CW. Testimony before the U.S. House of Representatives Committee on Small Business Subcommittee on Regulation, Business Opportunities, and Technology, Washington, DC, 10 November 1993. (See also Freundlich N. Birth control: Scared to a standstill—Most drugmakers dread the legal risks, so older methods still prevail. *Business Week*, 16 June 1997: 142–144).

7. Bangladesh, Brazil, China, Colombia, Dominican Republic, Ecuador, Egypt, Haiti, Indonesia, Kenya, Mexico, Nepal, Nigeria, Peru, Philippines, Rwanda, Sri Lanka, Thailand, United States, and Zambia.

8. Bahrain, Bangladesh, Burkina Faso, Canada, Chile, China, Colombia, Costa Rica, Cyprus, Czech Republic, Denmark, Dominican Republic, Ecuador, Egypt, Ethiopia, Finland, France, Germany, Ghana, Greece, Haiti, Indonesia, Iran, Israel, Jamaica, Kenya, Kuwait, Luxembourg, Madagascar, Malawi, Malaysia, Mali, Mauritius, Mexico, Nepal, Netherlands, Pakistan, Palau, Peru, Philippines, Romania, Rwanda, Senegal, Singapore, South Africa, Soviet Union (former), Sri Lanka, Sweden, Switzerland, Taiwan, Tanzania, Thailand, Tunisia, United Kingdom, United States, Venezuela, Zambia, Zimbabwe.

9. Kolata G. Will the lawyers kill off Norplant? After breast implants, American Home Products' birth-control device is this year's target. *New York Times*, 28 May 1995.

10. The agency published that affirmation in a *Talk Paper* of 17 August 1995, in which it announced approval of a new form incorporated into the product's labeling that allows patients to acknowledge receipt of information and the opportunity for thorough discussion regarding Norplant prior to insertion. It also reported that "The agency's ongoing analysis of adverse reaction reports and postmarketing surveillance studies had found no basis for questioning the safety and effectiveness of Norplant when used as directed in the labeling, noting that its review had already assessed the safety and effectiveness of the hormone

APPENDIX B

levonorgestrel for long-term contraception, as well as the safety of Norplant's silicone-based delivery system" (Food and Drug Administration. FDA Talk Paper. Rockville, MD: DHHS/PHS, 17 August 1995).

Also in 1995, in connection with the breast implant controversy, then-FDA Commissioner Kessler stated:

"One specific area where biological effects [of silicone] have been assessed is with the contraceptive implant, Norplant. This product is a piece of closed tubing of silicone elastomer filled with crystals . . . that deliver the drug over a five-year period. The biological safety of the tubing has been studied in laboratory and animal toxicity tests. The silicone materials caused the expected local reactions, but tests to detect immunologic reactions were negative. In addition, reported cases of autoimmune or potentially immune-related disorders among women using Norplant are consistent with the expected rate in this population" Federal Document Clearinghouse. Testimony by David A. Kessler, M.D., Commissioner, Food and Drug Administration: Congressional Testimony before the Subcommittee on Human Resources and Intergovernmental Relations, Committee on Governmental Reform and Oversight, U.S. House of Representatives, Washington, D.C., 1 August 1995.

11. *The Economist*. On the needless hounding of a safe contraceptive, 2 September 1995; Freundlich, op. cit., 1997.

12. One-third of the Norplant suits against American Home Products and its subsidiary, Wyeth Laboratories, Inc., were brought in state courts, principally in Texas, Illinois, and Indiana. Two-thirds were pending in federal courts and were consolidated for pretrial purposes in the U.S. District Court in Beaumont, Texas, as master class action complaint MDL 1038, on counts of strict products liability, negligence, breach of implied warranty of merchantability, misrepresentation, and consumer fraud.

In January 1995, Wyeth-Ayerst announced plans to "offer health care providers defense and indemnification in connection with claims and lawsuits associated with the Norplant system" as long as the contraceptive was prescribed, inserted, or removed according to labeling (F-D-C Reports. In Brief: Norplant. *Pink Sheet* 57(5):19, 1995).

In August 1996, U.S. District Court Judge Richard A. Schell, decided that class certification was premature and ordered three bellwether trials, each involving five plaintiffs, to aid the court in determining the appropriateness of issue certification for a nationwide class of plaintiffs. In the first bellwether suit in February 1997, Judge Schell denied claims that Wyeth had failed to adequately warn or disclose the severity of Norplant's potential side effects, either to consumers or prescribing physicians, and dismissed plaintiffs' claims of negligence and breach of warranty. In issuing its ruling, the court applied the learned intermediary doctrine, which holds that when a manufacturer sells a drug that is properly prepared and accompanied by proper directions and warnings to the prescribing physician (the "learned intermediary"), the drug is not viewed as defective or unreasonably dangerous and the manufacturer is neither liable for resulting damages nor responsible for warning each patient directly (RA Schell. *Memorandum Opinion and Order Granting Defendant's [Wyeth's] Motion for Summary Judgment*. U.S. District Court for the Eastern District of Texas, Beaumont Division, 3 March 1997; Nutton MB. Norplant litigation—Creating an exception to the learned intermediary doctrine. *Trial* 32(7):74–77, 1996). State courts in Illinois, Pennsylvania, and New Jersey have denied similar motions involving Norplant, and an Illinois court has also decertified a class of plaintiffs alleging removal difficulties (*Mealey's Litigation Report: Drugs and Medical Devices*. American Home updates pending Norplant suits. 18 April 1997).

On August 8, 1997, the Texas Supreme Court issued an order indefinitely delaying the trial set for August 11 that was to hear the suits brought by eight Texas women against Wyeth-Ayerst. The case was delayed so that the court could consider a motion by Wyeth attorneys to have several plaintiffs' attorneys disqualified for alleged misconduct (Court delays trial's start in Norplant case, *Houston Chronicle*, 8 August 1997, online http://www.chron.com/content/chron...politan/97/08/09/norplant.2-0.html).

13. In February 1996, Huhtamaki Oy announced negotiations on the sale of its pharmaceutical division, Leiras, to Schering AG. No allusion was made to Norplant as a factor in that decision. In fact, Norplant was part of the Schering purchase and Leiras has indicated that it intends to manufacture and market the two-rod implant system, under the name Jadelle® and outside the United States (S Waldman, personal communication, 20 August 1997).

C

Workshop Agenda

Implant Contraceptives:
An Illuminating Case Study in Current Dilemmas and Possibilities
7–8 April 1997

Objectives:

1. to review newly available data
2. to consider important ancillary issues
3. to extract generic lessons from a specific case
4. to explore preemptive approaches and mechanisms for introducing new contraceptives in the future

---

DAY ONE—MONDAY, 7 APRIL 1997

8:30 a.m. **OPENING STATEMENT, CHARGE TO COMMITTEE, PARTICIPANTS**
Allan Rosenfield, Chair

8:45 **WHAT INTERNATIONAL DATA TELL US NOW:**
(Committee Rapporteur: Hedia Belhadj)
Data and Analysis from WHO/HRP, Family Health International, and Population Council
Postmarketing Surveillance
Olav Meirik, WHO/HRP
Paul Van Look, WHO/HRP

QUESTIONS AND COMMENTS

10:00 **WHAT U.S. DATA TELL US NOW:**
(Committee Rapporteur: Nancy Buc)
Data and Analysis: NICHD and Kaiser-Funded Clinic-Based Studies
Andrew Davidson, Columbia University
Debra Kalmuss, Columbia University

10:30 *Helen Koo, Research Triangle Institute*

11:00 Data and Analysis from 1995 National Survey of Family Growth
Jacqueline Darroch, Alan Guttmacher Institute

11:30 Data and Analysis from Population Council Studies
Irving Sivin, Population Council

12 noon **QUESTIONS AND COMMENTS**

12:15 p.m. LUNCH

1:00 **A RANGE OF PERSPECTIVES: SOME PREPARED REMARKS AND A DIALOGUE**
(Committee Rapporteur: Rebecca Cook)
Cynthia Pearson, National Women's Health Network
Julia Scott, National Black Women's Health Project
Ellen Moskowitz, Hastings Center
Martha Ellen Katz, Department of Social Medicine, Harvard Medical School; Martha Eliot Health Center, Children's Hospital

QUESTIONS AND COMMENTS

2:30 **IMPLANT REMOVAL AND TRAINING**
(Committee Rapporteur: Judy Norsigian)

Clinical Issues:
David Archer, Eastern Virginia Medical/Jones Institute

Case Material:
United Kingdom:
Angela Davey, Hoechst-Marion-Roussel, United Kingdom with Lynne Gaffikin, JHPIEGO
Baltimore:
Paul Blumenthal, Johns Hopkins Bayview Medical Center
Indonesia:
Paul Blumenthal
Ruth Simmons, University of Michigan

METHOD COST-EFFECTIVENESS: IMPLICATIONS FOR NEW FORMULATIONS
(Committee Rapporteur: David Mowery)
Felicia Stewart, Kaiser Family Foundation

QUESTIONS AND COMMENTS

BREAK *ad libitum*

APPENDIX C 117

3:30 **BIOCOMPATIBILITY, MEDICAL APPLICATIONS OF SILICONE-BASED MATERIALS: REVIEW OF PERTINENT FINDINGS**
(Committee Rapporteur: Donald McDonnell)
James Anderson, Case Western Reserve
Noel Rose, Johns Hopkins

VAGINAL HIV/SIV TRANSMISSION
Monkey SIV Data:
Preston Marx, Aaron Diamond Research Center
Human Epidemiologic Data:
Ward Cates, Family Health International

QUESTIONS AND COMMENTS

5:30 **CHAIRMAN'S INSTRUCTIONS, ADJOURNMENT**

DAY TWO—TUESDAY, 8 APRIL 1997

8:30 **SUMMATION: WHAT HAVE WE HEARD? WHERE DOES IT LEAVE US?**

9:00 **LOOKING TO THE FUTURE**
A Federal Standards Defense: What Difference Might It Make?
Michael Green, Iowa Law Center

The Reproductive Health Technologies Project: Objectives and Plans
Marie Bass, Bass and Howes, Inc.

WHO Strategic Initiative for Introduction of New Methods: Illumination from Early Experience
Ruth Simmons

9:45 **OTHER PREPARATORY AND PREVENTIVE APPROACHES**
Lead Discussants:
Ruth Macklin, Albert Einstein College of Medicine
Marian Secundy, Howard University Program in Clinical Ethics

GENERAL DISCUSSION
Tutti

12:30 p.m. **ADJOURNMENT**

NATIONAL ACADEMY OF SCIENCES
INSTITUTE OF MEDICINE

WORKSHOP
Implant Contraceptives:
An Illuminating Case Study in Current Dilemmas and Possibilities

7 April 1997—Lecture Room
8 April 1997—Members' Room
2101 Constitution Avenue, N.W.
Washington, DC 20418

PARTICIPANTS

James M. Anderson, MD, PhD
Professor of Pathology,
    Macromolecular Science, and
    Biomedical Engineering
Case Western Reserve University

Lisa Angerame
Government Relations Manager
American Society for Reproductive
    Medicine
Washington, D.C.

Felice Apter, PhD
Research Division
Office of Population
U.S. Agency for International
    Development

David Archer, MD
Director of Clinical Research
The Jones Institute
Eastern Virgina Medical College

Marie Bass
Project Director
Reproductive Health Technologies
    Project
Washington, D.C.

Paul Blumenthal, MD
Associate Professor
Johns Hopkins University
Bayview Medical Center

Willard Cates, Jr., MD, MPH
Senior Vice President
Biomedical Affairs
Family Health International

Jacqueline E. Darroch, PhD
Senior Vice President
Vice President for Research
The Alan Guttmacher Institute

Angela Davey
Head, Medical Information Services
Hoechst Marion Roussel Ltd.
United Kingdom

Andrew R. Davidson, PhD, MBA
Center for Population
    and Family Health
Columbia University

Judith M. DeSarno
President and CEO
National Family Planning and
    Reproductive Health Association
Washington, D.C.

APPENDIX C 119

Henry L. Gabelnick, PhD
Director
Contraceptive Research and
 Development Program

Lynne Gaffikin, PhD
JHPIEGO Corporation
Baltimore, MD

Michael D. Green, JD
College of Law
University of Iowa

Gary Grubb, MD, MPH
Director
Women's Health Care
Wyeth Ayerst Laboratories

Diane Harrison, MD, FACOG
Director, Clinical Affairs
Medical Affairs Department
Wyeth-Ayerst Laboratories

Stephen F. Heartwell, MD
Associate Professor
Department of Obstetrics and
 Gynecology
University of Texas Southwestern
 Medical School
(Chair, Norplant Foundation)

Stephen Isaacs, JD
Center for Health and Social Policy
Pelham, New York

Lisa Kaeser
The Alan Guttmacher Institute
Washington, D.C.

Debra Kalmuss, PhD
Center for Population
 and Family Health
Columbia University

Martha Ellen Katz, MD
Department of Social Medicine
Harvard Medical School
Martha Eliot Health Center
Children's Hospital

Helen P. Koo, PhD
Research Triangle Institute

Johanna K. Kouru
General Counsel
Leiras Oy

Pekka Lahteenmaki, MD
Leiras Oy

Ruth Macklin, PhD
Professor
Department of Epidemiology
 and Social Medicine
Albert Einstein College of Medicine

Preston A. Marx, PhD
Aaron Diamond AIDS
 Research Center
AIDS Animal Models Laboratory
 at LEMSIP

Christine Mauck, MD
Medical Officer
Reproductive and Urologic Drug
 Products Division
Center for Drug Evaluation
 and Research
Food and Drug Administration

Olav Meirik, MD, PhD
Special Program of Research,
 Development, and
 Research Training in
 Human Reproduction
World Health Organization

Thomas Merrick
Advisor for Population
Human Development Department
The World Bank

Ellen Moskowitz, JD
Associate for Law
The Hastings Center

Susan F. Newcomer, PhD
Sociologist/Demographer
Demographic and Behavioral
　Sciences Branch
Center for Population Research
National Institute for Child Health
　and Human Development

Cynthia Pearson
Executive Director
National Women's Health Network

Marjorie Powell, JD
Assistant General Counsel
Pharmaceutical Research and
　Manufacturers Association

Noel Rose, MD, PhD
Professor
Department of Immunology
　and Infectious Disease
School of Hygiene
　and Public Health
Professor of Medicine
Johns Hopkins University

Julia R. Scott, RN
National Black Women's
　Health Network
Washington, D.C.

Marian Gray Secundy, EdD
Director, Program in Clinical Ethics
Department of Community Health
　and Family Practice
Howard University
College of Medicine

James Shelton, MD
Acting Chief
Office of Population
Bureau of Science and Technology
U.S. Agency for International
　Development

Ruth Simmons, PhD
Health Behavior and
　Health Education
School of Public Health
University of Michigan

Irving Sivin
Center for Biomedical Research
The Population Council

Jeffrey Spieler
Chief, Research Division
Office of Population
U.S. Agency for International
　Development

Robert Spirtas, DrPH
Chief
Contraceptive Evaluation Branch
Center for Population Research
National Institute of Child Health
　and Human Development

Felicia H. Stewart, MD
Director of Reproductive Health
　Programs
Henry J. Kaiser Family Foundation

Sean B. Tipton
Director of Public Affairs
The Endocrine Society

Paul Van Look, MD, PhD
Special Program of Research,
　Development, and Research
　Training in Human
　Reproduction
World Health Organization

Sandra Waldman, MA, MS
Director
Office of Public Information
The Population Council

Margaret Weber, MD
Senior Director, Clinical Affairs
Medical Affairs Department
Wyeth-Ayerst Laboratories